DSM-IV™
CODING UPDATE

1996 EDITION

Includes ICD-9-CM Codes
Effective October 1, 1996

Prepared by

Michael B. First, M.D.

Laurie E. McQueen, M.S.S.W.

Harold Alan Pincus, M.D.

Published by the American Psychiatric Association
Washington, D.C.

Copyright © 1996 American Psychiatric Association
ALL RIGHTS RESERVED
Manufactured in the United States of America on acid-free paper
First Edition
99 98 97 96   4 3 2 1

American Psychiatric Association
1400 K Street, N.W., Washington, DC   20005

Library of Congress Cataloging-in-Publication Data
First, Michael B., 1956–
    DSM-IV coding update / prepared by Michael B. First, Laurie E.
McQueen, Harold Alan Pincus.
        p.   cm.
    "1996 edition—includes ICD-9-CM codes effective October 1, 1996."
    Updates DSM-IV published in 1994.
    ISBN 0-89042-409-8
    1. Mental illness—Classification.   2. Mental illness—Diagnosis.
 I. McQueen, Laurie E.   II. Pincus, Harold Alan, 1951–   .
III. Diagnostic and statistical manual of mental disorders.
IV. Title.
    [DNLM: 1. Mental Disorders—classification.   2. Mental Disorders—
diagnosis.   WM 15 F527d 1997]
RC455.2.C4F57   1997
616.89′075—dc20
DNLM/DLC
for Library of Congress   96-38257
                                                                                            CIP

British Library Cataloguing in Publication Data
A CIP record is available from the British Library.

Contents

Introduction

The diagnostic codes in DSM-IV are an integral element of the system and are important for record keeping, data collection, communication, and reimbursement. It is therefore crucial that the codes be as accurate, up-to-date, and useful as possible. The official coding system currently in use in the United States is the International Classification of Diseases, Ninth Revision, Clinical Modification (ICD-9-CM). The use of the ICD-9-CM diagnostic codes has been mandated by the Health Care Financing Administration for purposes of reimbursement under the Medicare system. Other government agencies as well as most third-party payers also require these diagnostic codes for data collection and reimbursement purposes. To facilitate the use of DSM-IV in clinical and research settings, all of the diagnostic codes in DSM-IV have been selected from the ICD-9-CM system.

To keep the ICD-9-CM system up-to-date, changes are made to the system on a yearly basis, taking effect each October. This updating process is conducted by the ICD-9-CM Coordination and Maintenance Committee, a federal committee co-chaired by representatives of the National Center for Health Statistics (NCHS) and the Health Care Financing Administration (HCFA). Proposals for coding changes are submitted by professional organizations, industry groups, individual clinicians, and other interested parties, usually for the purpose of increasing coding specificity. Following a period of public comment, the committee submits its recommendations for changes to the diagnostic codes to the director of HCFA for final approval. The final coding changes are published as an Interim Final Notice in the May–June *Federal Register.*

When DSM-IV was published in May 1994, all of the diagnostic codes were compatible with the version of ICD-9-CM that was current at the time. However, since then, 2 years of coding revisions have gone into effect, with an additional set of changes to become effective as of October 1, 1996. There are two types of coding changes: 1) new diagnostic codes that are being added to the ICD-9-CM system, and 2) existing diagnostic codes that have become out-of-date and will no longer be accepted as legitimate codes. For inpatient hospital bills submitted to HCFA, use of the new codes becomes mandatory as of October 1, 1996. For physician bills submitted to HCFA, use of the new codes is not mandatory until

January 1, 1997. It should be noted that these effective dates apply only to diagnostic codes submitted to HCFA; other third-party payers might adopt other effective dates for these new codes.

This *Coding Update* is being published by the American Psychiatric Association with the goal of facilitating the incorporation of these new codes into DSM-IV. In addition, this update includes a few coding changes resulting from the identification of incorrect classification assignments in DSM-IV. The *Coding Update* is divided into three sections. Section I of the *Coding Update* provides an overall summary of the relevant ICD-9-CM coding changes that impact the DSM-IV Classification. It also includes changes in the diagnostic codes for those selected general medical conditions that appear in Appendix G of DSM-IV. Some people may wish to cut these pages out and paste them into their copy of DSM-IV (for example, the box showing changes to the Classification could be affixed to page 12 of DSM-IV, and the box showing changes to Appendix G could be affixed to the bottom of page 812). Section II presents the coding changes in an alternative format, indicating each page of DSM-IV on which there is a coding change. This format is useful for manually updating your copy of DSM-IV on a page-by-page basis. Section III provides answers to a number of the most commonly asked questions about DSM-IV and coding. Finally, Section IV includes updated versions incorporating the coding changes of those sections of DSM-IV that are most often used for coding purposes: the DSM-IV Classification (DSM-IV pages 13–24), Appendix E (Alphabetical Listing of DSM-IV Diagnoses and Codes; pages 793–802), Appendix F (Numerical Listing of DSM-IV Diagnoses and Codes; pages 803–812), and Appendix G (ICD-9-CM Codes for Selected General Medical Conditions and Medication-Induced Disorders; pages 813–828).

Section I

Summary of Changes

The following two pages provide a summary of the coding changes in DSM-IV. All diagnostic codes are effective for Federal Government reporting purposes as of October 1, 1996.

Feel free to cut and paste the box showing changes to the Classification to page 12 of DSM-IV, and the box showing changes to Appendix G to the bottom of page 812.

■ Coding Changes to DSM-IV Appendix G—Codes for Selected General Medical Conditions and Medication-Induced Disorders

Note: An asterisk (*) following the diagnostic code indicates that greater specificity is available. Refer to the ICD-9-CM Diseases: Tabular List (Volume 1) entry for that code for additional information.

414.00* Atherosclerotic heart disease *(former code: 414.0)*

415.19* Embolism, pulmonary *(former code: 415.1)*

278.00* Obesity *(former code: 278.0)*

575.11 Cholecystitis, chronic *(former code: 575.1)*

556.9* Colitis, ulcerative *(former code: 556)*

752.51 Undescended testicle *(former code: 752.5)*

042 HIV infection (symptomatic) *(former codes: 042.0–044.0)*

Section II

Coding Changes by Page

The following list indicates for which pages in DSM-IV there are coding changes. You can use this guide to update your version of DSM-IV with the new codes on a page-by-page basis. The locations (page and line number) of all obsolete codes are noted, and updated codes are provided.

p. 13, column 2, line 23, **change** 315.31 Mixed Receptive-Expressive Language Disorder **to** 315.32

p. 14, column 1, line 17, **replace**

312.8	Conduct Disorder
	Specify type: Childhood-Onset Type/Adolescent-Onset Type **with**
312.xx	Conduct Disorder
.81	Childhood-Onset Type
.82	Adolescent-Onset Type
.89	Unspecified Onset

p. 15, column 1, line 16, **change** 294.9 Dementia Due to HIV Disease **to** 294.1

p. 15, column 1, line 17, **change** *(also code 043.1 HIV infection affecting central nervous system on Axis III)* **to** *(also code 042 HIV infection on Axis III)*

p. 16, column 1, line 22, **change** 291.8 Alcohol Withdrawal **to** 291.81

p. 16, column 1, line 34, **change** 291.8 Alcohol-Induced Mood Disorder **to** 291.89

p. 16, column 1, line 36, **change** 291.8 Alcohol-Induced Anxiety Disorder **to** 291.89

p. 16, column 1, line 38, **change** 291.8 Alcohol-Induced Sexual Dysfunction **to** 291.89

p. 16, column 1, line 41, **change** 291.8 Alcohol-Induced Sleep Disorder **to** 291.89

p. 18, column 1, line 21, **change** 304.90 Phencyclidine Dependence **to** 304.60

p. 20, column 2, line 43, **change** 293.89 Anxiety Disorder Due to . . . **to** 293.84

p. 21, column 1, line 15, **change** 300.81 Undifferentiated Somatoform Disorder **to** 300.82

p. 21, column 1, line 33, **change** 300.81 Somatoform Disorder NOS **to** 300.82

p. 24, column 1, line 27, **change** V61.1 Partner Relational Problem **to** V61.10

p. 24, column 1, line 33, **change** *(code 995.5 if focus of attention is on victim)* **to** *(code 995.54 if focus of attention is on victim)*

p. 24, column 1, line 36, **change** *(code 995.5 if focus of attention is on victim)* **to** *(code 995.53 if focus of attention is on victim)*

p. 24, column 1, line 39, **change** *(code 995.5 if focus of attention is on victim)* **to** *(code 995.52 if focus of attention is on victim)*

p. 24, column 1, line 41, **replace with**
Physical Abuse of Adult
V61.12 (if by partner)
V62.83 (if by person other than partner)

p. 24, column 1, line 44, **replace with**
Sexual Abuse of Adult
V61.12 (if by partner)
V62.83 (if by person other than partner)

p. 24, column 1, line 45, **change** *(code 995.81 if focus of attention is on victim)* **to** *(code 995.83 if focus of attention is on victim)*

p. 33, line 28, **change** V61.1 Partner Relational Problem **to** V61.10

p. 35, line 24, **change** V61.1 Partner Relational Problem **to** V61.10

p. 58, after criteria box, line 1, **change** 315.31 Mixed Receptive-Expressive Language Disorder **to** 315.32

p. 59, top of page header, **change** 315.31 Mixed Receptive-Expressive Language Disorder **to** 315.32

p. 60, criteria box at bottom of page, line 1, **change** 315.31 Mixed Receptive-Expressive Language Disorder **to** 315.32

p. 61, criteria box at top of page, line 1, **change** 315.31 Mixed Receptive-Expressive Language Disorder *(continued)* **to** 315.32

p. 85, top of page header, 312.8 Conduct Disorder, **delete** 312.8 and leave blank

p. 85, after criteria box, line 5, 312.8 Conduct Disorder, **delete** code 312.8 and leave blank

p. 86, line 39, **add** 312.81 before Childhood-Onset Type

p. 87, top of page header, 312.8 Conduct Disorder, **delete** 312.8 and leave blank

p. 87, line 1, **add** 312.82 before Adolescent-Onset Type

p. 87, after paragraph describing Adolescent-Onset Type, **add**
> **312.89**   **Unspecified Onset.** This code is used if the onset of Conduct Disorder is unknown.

p. 89, top of page header, 312.8 Conduct Disorder, **delete** 312.8 and leave blank

p. 90, criteria box, line 1, Diagnostic criteria for 312.8 Conduct Disorder, **delete** code 312.8 and leave blank

p. 91, criteria box, line 1, Diagnostic criteria for 312.8 Conduct Disorder *(continued),* **delete** code 312.8 and leave blank

p. 91, criteria box, **delete** lines 6–10 and **replace with** the following:
Code based on type:
> **312.81**   **Conduct Disorder, Childhood-Onset Type:** onset of at least one criterion characteristic of Conduct Disorder prior to age 10 years
> **312.82**   **Conduct Disorder, Adolescent-Onset Type:** absence of any criteria characteristic of Conduct Disorder prior to age 10 years
> **312.89**   **Conduct Disorder, Unspecified Onset:** age at onset is not known

p. 148, line 1, **change** 294.9 Dementia Due to HIV Disease **to** 294.1

p. 152, criteria box, line 7, **change** 294.9 Dementia Due to HIV Disease **to** 294.1

p. 152, criteria box, line 8, **replace** Coding note: Also code 043.1 HIV infection affecting central nervous system on Axis III. **with Coding note:** Also code 042 HIV infection on Axis III.

p. 166, line 14, **change** 293.89 Anxiety Disorder Due to a General Medical Condition **to** 293.84

p. 195, line 10, **change** 291.8 Alcohol Withdrawal **to** 291.81

p. 195, line 19, **change** 291.8 Alcohol-Induced Mood Disorder **to** 291.89

p. 195, line 21, **change** 291.8 Alcohol-Induced Anxiety Disorder **to** 291.89

p. 195, line 23, **change** 291.8 Alcohol-Induced Sexual Dysfunction **to** 291.89

p. 195, line 25, **change** 291.8 Alcohol-Induced Sleep Disorder **to** 291.89

p. 197, after criteria box, line 1, **change** 291.8 Alcohol Withdrawal **to** 291.81

p. 198, criteria box, line 1, **change** Diagnostic criteria for 291.8 Alcohol Withdrawal **to** 291.81

p. 199, criteria box, line 1, **change** Diagnostic criteria for 291.8 Alcohol Withdrawal *(continued)* **to** 291.81

p. 256, line 9, **change** 304.90 Phencyclidine Dependence **to** 304.60

p. 256, line 25, **change** 304.90 Phencyclidine Dependence **to** 304.60

p. 375, criteria box, line 4, **change** 291.8 Alcohol **to** 291.89

p. 436, after criteria box, line 1, **change** 293.89 Anxiety Disorder Due to a General Medical Condition **to** 293.84

p. 437, top of page header, **change** 293.89 Anxiety Disorder Due to General Medical Condition **to** 293.84

p. 437, line 41, **change** 293.89 Anxiety Disorder Due to Thyrotoxicosis, With Generalized Anxiety **to** 293.84

p. 439, criteria box, line 1, **change** Diagnostic criteria for 293.89 Anxiety Disorder Due to . . . *[Indicate the General Medical Condition]* **to** 293.84

p. 439, criteria box, line 23, **change** 293.89 Anxiety Disorder Due to Pheochromocytoma **to** 293.84

p. 441, line 18, **change** 291.8 Alcohol-Induced Anxiety Disorder **to** 291.89

p. 443, criteria box, line 31, **change** 291.8 Alcohol **to** 291.89

p. 450, after criteria box, line 1, **change** 300.81 Undifferentiated Somatoform Disorder **to** 300.82

p. 451, top of page header, **change** 300.81 Undifferentiated Somatoform Disorder **to** 300.82

p. 451, criteria box, line 1, **change** Diagnostic criteria for 300.81 Undifferentiated Somatoform Disorder **to** 300.82

p. 452, criteria box, line 1, **change** Diagnostic criteria for 300.81 Undifferentiated Somatoform Disorder *(continued)* **to** 300.82

p. 468, after criteria box, line 1, **change** 300.81 Somatoform Disorder Not Otherwise Specified **to** 300.82

p. 469, top of page header, **change** 300.81 Somatoform Disorder Not Otherwise Specified **to** 300.82

p. 520, line 12, **change** 291.8 Alcohol-Induced Sexual Dysfunction **to** 291.89

p. 522, criteria box, line 12, **change** 291.8 Alcohol **to** 291.89

p. 603, line 15, **change** 291.8 Alcohol-Induced Sleep Disorder **to** 291.89

p. 607, criteria box, line 23, **change** 291.8 Alcohol **to** 291.89

p. 681, line 14, **change** V61.1 Partner Relational Problem **to** V61.10

p. 682, **delete** line 8, **replace with** "the victim of the abuse or neglect, code 995.52, 995.53, or 995.54 for a child or 995.81 or 995.83 for an adult (depending on the type of abuse)"

p. 682, **delete** line 12, **replace with** the following:
Coding note: Specify **995.54** *if focus of clinical attention is on the victim.*

p. 682, **delete** line 16, **replace with** the following:
Coding note: Specify **995.53** *if focus of clinical attention is on the victim.*

p. 682, **delete** line 19, **replace with** the following:
Coding note: Specify **995.52** *if focus of clinical attention is on the victim.*

p. 682, line 20, **delete** V61.1 Physical Abuse of Adult and leave blank

p. 682, **delete** line 23, and **replace with** the following:
Coding note: Specify **V61.12** *if focus of clinical attention is on the perpetrator and abuse is by partner,* **V62.83** *if focus of clinical attention is on the perpetrator and abuse is by person other than partner,* **995.81** *if focus of clinical attention is on the victim.*

p. 682, line 24, **delete** V61.1 Sexual Abuse of Adult and leave blank

p. 682, **delete** line 27, **replace with** the following:
Coding note: Specify **V61.12** *if focus of clinical attention is on the perpetrator and abuse is by partner,* **V62.83** *if focus of clinical attention is on the perpetrator and abuse is by person other than partner,* **995.83** *if focus of clinical attention is on the victim.*

p. 726, line 4, **change** Physical Abuse of Child (995.5) **to** 995.54

p. 793, line 23, **change** 291.8 -Induced Anxiety Disorder **to** 291.89

p. 793, line 24, **change** 291.8 -Induced Mood Disorder **to** 291.89

p. 793, line 30, **change** 291.8 -Induced Sexual Dysfunction **to** 291.89

p. 793, line 31, **change** 291.8 -Induced Sleep Disorder **to** 291.89

p. 794, line 5, **change** 291.8 Withdrawal **to** 291.81

p. 794, line 25, **change** 293.89 Anxiety Disorder Due to . . . *[Indicate the General Medical Condition]* **to** 293.84

p. 796, line 17, 312.8 Conduct Disorder, **delete** 312.8; after line 17, **add** the following:
312.81 Childhood-Onset Type
312.82 Adolescent-Onset Type
312.89 Unspecified Onset

p. 796, line 25, **change** 294.9 Dementia Due to HIV Disease **to** 294.1

p. 798, line 48, **change** 315.31 Mixed Receptive-Expressive Language Disorder **to** 315.32

p. 799, line 6, **change** 995.5 Neglect of Child *(if focus of attention is on victim)* **to** 995.52

p. 800, line 21, **change** V61.1 Partner Relational Problem **to** V61.10

p. 800, line 30, **change** 304.90 Phencyclidine Dependence **to** 304.60

p. 800, **replace** line 40 **with** V61.12 Physical Abuse of Adult (if by partner)

p. 800, after line 40, **add** V62.83 Physical Abuse of Adult (if by person other than partner)

p. 800, line 43, **change** 995.5 Physical Abuse of Child *(if focus of attention is on victim)* **to** 995.54

p. 801, **replace** line 46 **with** V61.12 Sexual Abuse of Adult (if by partner)

p. 801, after line 46, **add** V62.83 Sexual Abuse of Adult (if by person other than partner)

p. 801, line 47, **change** 995.81 Sexual Abuse of Adult *(if focus of attention is on victim)* **to** 995.83

p. 801, line 49, **change** 995.5 Sexual Abuse of Child *(if focus of attention is on victim)* **to** 995.53

p. 802, line 17, **change** 300.81 Somatoform Disorder NOS **to** 300.82

p. 802, line 26, **change** 300.81 Undifferentiated Somatoform Disorder **to** 300.82

p. 803, after line 29, **add** 291.81 Alcohol Withdrawal

p. 803, line 30, **change** 291.8 Alcohol-Induced Anxiety Disorder **to** 291.89

p. 804, line 1, **change** 291.8 Alcohol-Induced Mood Disorder **to** 291.89

p. 804, line 2, **change** 291.8 Alcohol-Induced Sexual Dysfunction **to** 291.89

p. 804, line 3, **change** 291.8 Alcohol-Induced Sleep Disorder **to** 291.89

p. 804, **delete** line 4, 291.8 Alcohol Withdrawal

p. 806, line 6, **change** 293.89 Anxiety Disorder Due to . . . *[Indicate the General Medical Condition]* **to** 293.84

p. 806, after line 10, **add** 294.1 Dementia Due to HIV Disease

p. 806, **delete** line 14, 294.9 Dementia Due to HIV Disease

p. 808, line 14, **change** 300.81 Somatoform Disorder NOS **to** 300.82

p. 808, line 15, **change** 300.81 Undifferentiated Somatoform Disorder **to** 300.82

p. 809, after line 10, **add** 304.60 Phencyclidine Dependence

p. 809, **delete** line 13, 304.90 Phencyclidine Dependence

p. 810, line 23, **delete** 312.8 Conduct Disorder, **replace with** the following:
    312.81 Conduct Disorder, Childhood-Onset Type
    312.82 Conduct Disorder, Adolescent-Onset Type
    312.89 Conduct Disorder, Unspecified Onset

p. 810, line 39, **change** 315.31 Mixed Receptive-Expressive Language Disorder **to** 315.32

p. 811, line 36, **change** 995.5 Neglect of Child *(if focus of attention is on victim)* **to** 995.52

p. 811, after line 36, **add** 995.53 Sexual Abuse of Child *(if focus of attention is on victim)*

p. 811, line 37, **change** 995.5 Physical Abuse of Child *(if focus of attention is on victim)* **to** 995.54

p. 811, **delete** line 38, 995.5 Sexual Abuse of Child *(if focus of attention is on victim)*

p. 811, line 40, **change** 995.81 Sexual Abuse of Adult *(if focus of attention is on victim)* **to** 995.83

p. 811, line 42, **change** V61.1 Partner Relational Problem **to** V61.10

p. 811, line 43, **change** V61.1 Physical Abuse of Adult **to** V61.12 Physical Abuse of Adult (if by partner)

p. 811, line 44, **change** V61.1 Sexual Abuse of Adult **to** V61.12 Sexual Abuse of Adult (if by partner)

p. 812, after line 10, **add:**
V62.83   Physical Abuse of Adult (if by person other than partner)
V62.83   Sexual Abuse of Adult (if by person other than partner)

p. 815, line 35, **change** 414.0 Atherosclerotic heart disease **to** 414.00[*]

p. 815, line 44, **change** 415.1 Embolism, pulmonary **to** 415.19[*]

p. 819, line 9, **change** 278.0 Obesity **to** 278.00[*]

p. 819, line 43, **change** 575.1 Cholecystitis, chronic **to** 575.11

p. 820, line 1, **change** 556 Colitis, ulcerative **to** 556.9[*]

p. 823, line 23, **change** 752.5 Undescended testicle **to** 752.51

p. 823, **delete** lines 37–42

p. 824, after line 43, **add** 042 HIV infection (symptomatic)

p. 824, **delete** lines 1–13

Section III

Commonly Asked Questions About DSM-IV and Coding

Q. When should I start using the updated codes published in this coding update?

A. The updated diagnostic codes become "effective" October 1, 1996. For inpatients' Medicare reimbursement, the updated codes must be used for all discharge diagnoses submitted on or after October 1, 1996. For physician submissions, both the former codes and updated codes will be accepted from October 1, 1996, through December 31, 1996. Starting January 1, 1997, updated codes must be used for all physician reimbursement.

Q. Medicare, Medicaid, and other third-party payers require ICD-9-CM codes for diagnosis/reimbursement. Do I need a table to convert from DSM-IV codes to ICD-9-CM codes?

A. No. Unlike DSM-III and DSM-III-R, all of the diagnostic codes in DSM-IV were selected to be compatible with the version of ICD-9-CM that was current as of the publication of DSM-IV in May 1994. However, as discussed in the introduction (see page vii), the ICD-9-CM system is revised on a yearly basis, necessitating changes in the DSM-IV coding to keep it up-to-date. The *DSM-IV Coding Update* has been published to facilitate incorporation of these coding changes into your practice. Mental health organizations will be sent notices of these coding changes encouraging them to disseminate them to their members.

Q. Sometimes different disorders or subtypes of disorders have the same diagnostic code. Is this an error?

A. The DSM-IV diagnostic codes are limited to those contained within the ICD-9-CM coding system, which is required by most government agencies and private insurers. Like DSM-III and DSM-III-R, DSM-IV contains more diagnostic entities than there are official codes in ICD-9-CM. Therefore, by necessity, some DSM-IV diagnoses share diagnostic codes. Although this situation is certainly not optimal, it is necessary at times (particularly in coding substance-related disorders) to use the same code for more than one disorder.

Q. The lack of specific codes for subtypes and specifiers makes data collection sometimes difficult. Is there any way to get new, more specific codes put into DSM-IV so that every condition has its own unique code?

A. The ICD-9-CM Coordination and Maintenance Committee, a government agency, is charged with the task of maintaining the current diagnostic coding system and of making changes or additions to it. Virtually all of the available digits in the mental disorders section of ICD-9-CM have been used, leaving very few options for expansion of the codes. In developing DSM-IV, we considered providing a standardized system that would allow individual institutions to add a sixth digit to their local data systems to create greater specificity. However, it was decided that such action would increase the likelihood of reimbursements being rejected for incorrect codes; therefore, it was never adopted.

The American Psychiatric Association has proposed some new codes (which were ultimately approved by the ICD-9-CM Coordination and Maintenance Committee), and we are continuing to explore options for instituting additional new codes (for example, in response to numerous requests from researchers and clinicians, we are proposing a new fifth-digit coding assignment for the "with behavioral disturbance" specifier that would apply to Dementia of the Alzheimer's Type and Vascular Dementia).

Q. Are there any plans to develop a DSM-IV-R?

A. No. However, because DSM-IV has become widely used as a textbook, it is important that the data in the text sections, like other textbooks, be kept up-to-date. A text revision of DSM-IV is planned for publication in 1999/2000. No changes to the diagnostic categories or the criteria sets will be made. The only changes will be to update those text sections that provide information regarding prevalence, course, associated features, and so on.

Q. Has the *DSM-IV Sourcebook* been published yet?

A. Volume 1 of the *DSM-IV Sourcebook* (which contains literature reviews on substance-related disorders; delirium, dementia, and amnestic and other cognitive disorders; schizophrenia and other psychotic disorders; medication-induced movement disorders; and sleep disorders) was published in 1994. Volume 2 of the *Sourcebook* also is now available through American Psychiatric Press and contains literature reviews on mood disorders, late luteal phase dysphoric disorder, anxiety disorders, personality disorders, psychiatric system interface disorders, and sexual disorders. Volume 3 will be published in Fall 1996. This volume presents literature reviews on disorders usually first diagnosed in infancy, childhood, or adolescence; eating disorders; the DSM-IV multiaxial system; family/relational problems; and cultural issues. The final volume of the *Sourcebook,* Volume 4, will contain the reports from the MacArthur Data Reanalysis, the reports from the NIMH-sponsored DSM-IV Field Trials, and final integrative summaries from each of the DSM-IV Work Groups. Volume 4 is slated for publication in Fall 1997.

Q. I understand that there is a primary care version of DSM-IV—please tell me about it.

A. In October 1995, the APA published the *Diagnostic and Statistical Manual of Mental Disorders, Fourth Edition—Primary Care Version* (DSM-IV–PC). The DSM-IV–PC was designed specifically for use by primary care clinicians. Those mental disorders and conditions most frequently encountered in primary care constitute the majority of the manual. These disorders are presented in nine algorithms (depressed mood, anxiety, unexplained physical symptoms, cognitive disturbance, problematic substance use, sexual dysfunction, sleep disorders, weight change/eating problems, and psychotic symptoms). The DSM-IV–PC also includes sections on psychosocial problems that are a focus of clinical attention but that are not considered mental disorders, disorders that are rarely first identified in primary care (e.g., dissociative disorders, psychotic disorders, and disorders usually first diagnosed in infancy, childhood, or adolescence). A DSM-IV–PC Coding Update, indicating changes to the diagnostic codes in the DSM-IV–PC, is available from the APA Office of Research.

Q. What is the status of ICD-10?

A. ICD-10, the tenth revision of the International Classification of Diseases, was published by the World Health Organization in 1993. Although DSM-IV was developed with the explicit goal of ICD-10 compatibility, it includes ICD-9-CM codes because implementation of ICD-10 in the United States has been significantly delayed. Currently, the National Center for Health Statistics is developing a modification of ICD-10 (to be known as ICD-10-CM) for use in the United States, which will be field-tested over the next several years. It is anticipated that it will be required for reporting purposes no earlier than the year 2000.

Q. As a psychiatrist working outside the United States, I need to use ICD-10 codes when diagnosing a patient. Is there a version of DSM-IV or other information that allows me to do this?

A. Yes. DSM-IV contains Appendix H, which provides the ICD-10 codes for all DSM-IV diagnoses. In addition, an International Version of DSM-IV is available for those psychiatrists in countries that use ICD-10. *DSM-IV: International Version* features ICD-10 codes and additional text sections describing the relationship between the DSM-IV criteria sets and the ICD-10 Diagnostic Criteria for Research.

Q. Whom do I contact if I find a mistake or inconsistency in DSM-IV?

A. The APA Office of Research has responsibility for correcting errors in DSM-IV. Please describe the problem, noting the page number in DSM-IV, and mail it to DSM Coordinator, Office of Research, American Psychiatric Association, 1400 K Street, N.W., Washington, D.C. 20005, or fax it to (202) 789-1874.

Q. How do I order copies of DSM-IV and the other publications mentioned here?

A. DSM-IV can be ordered from American Psychiatric Press, Inc. (APPI): toll-free phone line: (800) 368-5777; fax: (202) 789-2648; or e-mail: order@appi.org.

Section IV

Updates of DSM-IV Sections Most Often Used for Coding

This section includes updated versions incorporating the new codes of those sections of DSM-IV that are most often used for coding purposes: the DSM-IV Classification (DSM-IV pages 13–24), Appendix E (Alphabetical Listing of DSM-IV Diagnoses and Codes; pages 793–802), Appendix F (Numerical Listing of DSM-IV Diagnoses and Codes; pages 803–812), and Appendix G (ICD-9-CM Codes for Selected General Medical Conditions and Medication-Induced Disorders; pages 813–828).

DSM-IV Classification

Updated to include ICD-9-CM codes effective October 1, 1996

NOS = Not Otherwise Specified.

An *x* appearing in a diagnostic code indicates that a specific code number is required.

An ellipsis (. . .) is used in the names of certain disorders to indicate that the name of a specific mental disorder or general medical condition should be inserted when recording the name (e.g., 293.0 Delirium Due to Hypothyroidism).

Numbers in parentheses are page numbers.

If criteria are currently met, one of the following severity specifiers may be noted after the diagnosis:

> Mild
> Moderate
> Severe

If criteria are no longer met, one of the following specifiers may be noted:

> In Partial Remission
> In Full Remission
> Prior History

Disorders Usually First Diagnosed in Infancy, Childhood, or Adolescence (37)

MENTAL RETARDATION (39)

Note: *These are coded on Axis II.*

317	Mild Mental Retardation (41)
318.0	Moderate Mental Retardation (41)
318.1	Severe Mental Retardation (41)
318.2	Profound Mental Retardation (41)
319	Mental Retardation, Severity Unspecified (42)

LEARNING DISORDERS (46)

315.00	Reading Disorder (48)
315.1	Mathematics Disorder (50)
315.2	Disorder of Written Expression (51)
315.9	Learning Disorder NOS (53)

MOTOR SKILLS DISORDER

315.4	Developmental Coordination Disorder (53)

COMMUNICATION DISORDERS (55)

315.31	Expressive Language Disorder (55)
315.32	Mixed Receptive-Expressive Language Disorder (58)
315.39	Phonological Disorder (61)
307.0	Stuttering (63)
307.9	Communication Disorder NOS (65)

PERVASIVE DEVELOPMENTAL DISORDERS (65)

299.00	Autistic Disorder (66)
299.80	Rett's Disorder (71)

299.10 Childhood Disintegrative Disorder (73)

299.80 Asperger's Disorder (75)

299.80 Pervasive Developmental Disorder NOS (77)

ATTENTION-DEFICIT AND DISRUPTIVE BEHAVIOR DISORDERS (78)

314.xx Attention-Deficit/Hyperactivity Disorder (78)
   .01 Combined Type
   .00 Predominantly Inattentive Type
   .01 Predominantly Hyperactive-Impulsive Type

314.9 Attention-Deficit/Hyperactivity Disorder NOS (85)

312.xx Conduct Disorder (85)
   .81 Childhood-Onset Type
   .82 Adolescent-Onset Type
   .89 Unspecified Onset

313.81 Oppositional Defiant Disorder (91)

312.9 Disruptive Behavior Disorder NOS (94)

FEEDING AND EATING DISORDERS OF INFANCY OR EARLY CHILDHOOD (94)

307.52 Pica (95)

307.53 Rumination Disorder (96)

307.59 Feeding Disorder of Infancy or Early Childhood (98)

TIC DISORDERS (100)

307.23 Tourette's Disorder (101)

307.22 Chronic Motor or Vocal Tic Disorder (103)

307.21 Transient Tic Disorder (104)
Specify if: Single Episode/Recurrent

307.20 Tic Disorder NOS (105)

ELIMINATION DISORDERS (106)

—.– Encopresis (106)

787.6 With Constipation and Overflow Incontinence

307.7 Without Constipation and Overflow Incontinence

307.6 Enuresis (Not Due to a General Medical Condition) (108)
Specify type: Nocturnal Only/Diurnal Only/Nocturnal and Diurnal

OTHER DISORDERS OF INFANCY, CHILDHOOD, OR ADOLESCENCE

309.21 Separation Anxiety Disorder (110)
Specify if: Early Onset

313.23 Selective Mutism (114)

313.89 Reactive Attachment Disorder of Infancy or Early Childhood (116)
Specify type: Inhibited Type/Disinhibited Type

307.3 Stereotypic Movement Disorder (118)
Specify if: With Self-Injurious Behavior

313.9 Disorder of Infancy, Childhood, or Adolescence NOS (121)

Delirium, Dementia, and Amnestic and Other Cognitive Disorders (123)

DELIRIUM (124)

293.0 Delirium Due to . . . *[Indicate the General Medical Condition]* (127)

—.– Substance Intoxication Delirium *(refer to Substance-Related Disorders for substance-specific codes)* (129)

—.– Substance Withdrawal Delirium *(refer to Substance-Related Disorders for substance-specific codes)* (129)

—.– Delirium Due to Multiple Etiologies *(code each of the specific etiologies)* (132)

780.09 Delirium NOS (133)

DEMENTIA (133)

290.xx   Dementia of the Alzheimer's Type, With Early Onset *(also code 331.0 Alzheimer's disease on Axis III)* (139)

.10   Uncomplicated

.11   With Delirium

.12   With Delusions

.13   With Depressed Mood

Specify if: With Behavioral Disturbance

290.xx   Dementia of the Alzheimer's Type, With Late Onset *(also code 331.0 Alzheimer's disease on Axis III)* (139)

.0   Uncomplicated

.3   With Delirium

.20   With Delusions

.21   With Depressed Mood

Specify if: With Behavioral Disturbance

290.xx   Vascular Dementia (143)

.40   Uncomplicated

.41   With Delirium

.42   With Delusions

.43   With Depressed Mood

Specify if: With Behavioral Disturbance

294.1   Dementia Due to HIV Disease *(also code 042 HIV infection on Axis III)* (148)

294.1   Dementia Due to Head Trauma *(also code 854.00 head injury on Axis III)* (148)

294.1   Dementia Due to Parkinson's Disease *(also code 332.0 Parkinson's disease on Axis III)* (148)

294.1   Dementia Due to Huntington's Disease *(also code 333.4 Huntington's disease on Axis III)* (149)

290.10   Dementia Due to Pick's Disease *(also code 331.1 Pick's disease on Axis III)* (149)

290.10   Dementia Due to Creutzfeldt-Jakob Disease *(also code 046.1 Creutzfeldt-Jakob disease on Axis III)* (150)

294.1   Dementia Due to . . . *[Indicate the General Medical Condition not listed above] (also code the general medical condition on Axis III)* (151)

——.–   Substance-Induced Persisting Dementia *(refer to Substance-Related Disorders for substance-specific codes)* (152)

——.–   Dementia Due to Multiple Etiologies *(code each of the specific etiologies)* (154)

294.8   Dementia NOS (155)

AMNESTIC DISORDERS (156)

294.0   Amnestic Disorder Due to . . . *[Indicate the General Medical Condition]* (158)

Specify if: Transient/Chronic

——.–   Substance-Induced Persisting Amnestic Disorder *(refer to Substance-Related Disorders for substance-specific codes)* (161)

294.8   Amnestic Disorder NOS (163)

OTHER COGNITIVE DISORDERS (163)

294.9   Cognitive Disorder NOS (163)

Mental Disorders Due to a General Medical Condition Not Elsewhere Classified (165)

293.89   Catatonic Disorder Due to . . . *[Indicate the General Medical Condition]* (169)

310.1   Personality Change Due to . . . *[Indicate the General Medical Condition]* (171)

Specify type: Labile Type/ Disinhibited Type/Aggressive Type/Apathetic Type/Paranoid Type/Other Type/Combined Type/Unspecified Type

293.9   Mental Disorder NOS Due to . . . *[Indicate the General Medical Condition]* (174)

Substance-Related Disorders (175)

[a]*The following specifiers may be applied to Substance Dependence:*

With Physiological Dependence/
Without Physiological Dependence

Early Full Remission/Early Partial Remission
Sustained Full Remission/Sustained Partial
Remission
On Agonist Therapy/In a Controlled
Environment

The following specifiers apply to Substance-Induced Disorders as noted:
[I]With Onset During Intoxication/[W]With Onset
During Withdrawal

ALCOHOL-RELATED DISORDERS (194)
Alcohol Use Disorders
303.90 Alcohol Dependence[a] (195)
305.00 Alcohol Abuse (196)

Alcohol-Induced Disorders
303.00 Alcohol Intoxication (196)
291.81 Alcohol Withdrawal (197)
    Specify if: With Perceptual
    Disturbances
291.0   Alcohol Intoxication Delirium (129)
291.0   Alcohol Withdrawal Delirium (129)
291.2   Alcohol-Induced Persisting
        Dementia (152)
291.1   Alcohol-Induced Persisting Amnestic
        Disorder (161)
291.x   Alcohol-Induced Psychotic
        Disorder (310)
    .5   With Delusions[I,W]
    .3   With Hallucinations[I,W]
291.89 Alcohol-Induced Mood
        Disorder[I,W] (370)
291.89 Alcohol-Induced Anxiety
        Disorder[I,W] (439)
291.89 Alcohol-Induced Sexual
        Dysfunction[I] (519)
291.89 Alcohol-Induced Sleep
        Disorder[I,W] (601)

291.9   Alcohol-Related Disorder
        NOS (204)

AMPHETAMINE (OR AMPHETAMINE-LIKE)–RELATED DISORDERS (204)
Amphetamine Use Disorders
304.40 Amphetamine Dependence[a] (206)
305.70 Amphetamine Abuse (206)

Amphetamine-Induced Disorders
292.89 Amphetamine Intoxication (207)
    Specify if: With Perceptual
    Disturbances
292.0   Amphetamine Withdrawal (208)
292.81 Amphetamine Intoxication
        Delirium (129)
292.xx Amphetamine-Induced
        Psychotic Disorder (310)
    .11   With Delusions[I]
    .12   With Hallucinations[I]
292.84 Amphetamine-Induced Mood
        Disorder[I,W] (370)
292.89 Amphetamine-Induced Anxiety
        Disorder[I] (439)
292.89 Amphetamine-Induced Sexual
        Dysfunction[I] (519)
292.89 Amphetamine-Induced Sleep
        Disorder[I,W] (601)

292.9   Amphetamine-Related Disorder
        NOS (211)

CAFFEINE-RELATED DISORDERS (212)
Caffeine-Induced Disorders
305.90 Caffeine Intoxication (212)
292.89 Caffeine-Induced Anxiety Disorder[I]
        (439)
292.89 Caffeine-Induced Sleep
        Disorder[I] (601)

292.9   Caffeine-Related Disorder
        NOS (215)

CANNABIS-RELATED DISORDERS (215)
Cannabis Use Disorders
304.30 Cannabis Dependence[a] (216)
305.20 Cannabis Abuse (217)

Cannabis-Induced Disorders
292.89 Cannabis Intoxication (217)
    Specify if: With Perceptual
    Disturbances
292.81 Cannabis Intoxication
        Delirium (129)

292.xx   Cannabis-Induced Psychotic
　　　　Disorder (310)
　　.11　　With Delusions[I]
　　.12　　With Hallucinations[I]
292.89   Cannabis-Induced Anxiety
　　　　Disorder[I] (439)

292.9   Cannabis-Related Disorder
　　　　NOS (221)

COCAINE-RELATED DISORDERS (221)
Cocaine Use Disorders
304.20   Cocaine Dependence[a] (222)
305.60   Cocaine Abuse (223)

Cocaine-Induced Disorders
292.89   Cocaine Intoxication (223)
　　　　Specify if:　With Perceptual
　　　　Disturbances
292.0   Cocaine Withdrawal (225)
292.81   Cocaine Intoxication
　　　　Delirium (129)
292.xx   Cocaine-Induced Psychotic
　　　　Disorder (310)
　　.11　　With Delusions[I]
　　.12　　With Hallucinations[I]
292.84   Cocaine-Induced Mood Disorder[I,W]
　　　　(370)
292.89   Cocaine-Induced Anxiety
　　　　Disorder[I,W] (439)
292.89   Cocaine-Induced Sexual
　　　　Dysfunction[I] (519)
292.89   Cocaine-Induced Sleep Disorder[I,W]
　　　　(601)

292.9   Cocaine-Related Disorder
　　　　NOS (229)

HALLUCINOGEN-RELATED
DISORDERS (229)
Hallucinogen Use Disorders
304.50   Hallucinogen Dependence[a] (230)
305.30   Hallucinogen Abuse (231)

Hallucinogen-Induced Disorders
292.89   Hallucinogen Intoxication (232)
292.89   Hallucinogen Persisting Perception
　　　　Disorder (Flashbacks) (233)
292.81   Hallucinogen Intoxication Delirium
　　　　(129)

292.xx   Hallucinogen-Induced Psychotic
　　　　Disorder (310)
　　.11　　With Delusions[I]
　　.12　　With Hallucinations[I]
292.84   Hallucinogen-Induced Mood
　　　　Disorder[I] (370)
292.89   Hallucinogen-Induced Anxiety
　　　　Disorder[I] (439)

292.9   Hallucinogen-Related Disorder
　　　　NOS (236)

INHALANT-RELATED DISORDERS (236)
Inhalant Use Disorders
304.60   Inhalant Dependence[a] (238)
305.90   Inhalant Abuse (238)

Inhalant-Induced Disorders
292.89   Inhalant Intoxication (239)
292.81   Inhalant Intoxication
　　　　Delirium (129)
292.82   Inhalant-Induced Persisting
　　　　Dementia (152)
292.xx   Inhalant-Induced Psychotic
　　　　Disorder (310)
　　.11　　With Delusions[I]
　　.12　　With Hallucinations[I]
292.84   Inhalant-Induced Mood
　　　　Disorder[I] (370)
292.89   Inhalant-Induced Anxiety Disorder[I]
　　　　(439)

292.9   Inhalant-Related Disorder
　　　　NOS (242)

NICOTINE-RELATED DISORDERS (242)
Nicotine Use Disorder
305.10   Nicotine Dependence[a] (243)

Nicotine-Induced Disorder
292.0   Nicotine Withdrawal (244)

292.9   Nicotine-Related Disorder
　　　　NOS (247)

OPIOID-RELATED DISORDERS (247)
Opioid Use Disorders
304.00   Opioid Dependence[a] (248)
305.50   Opioid Abuse (249)

Opioid-Induced Disorders
292.89   Opioid Intoxication (249)
　　　　Specify if:　With Perceptual
　　　　Disturbances

292.0   Opioid Withdrawal (250)

292.81   Opioid Intoxication Delirium (129)

292.xx   Opioid-Induced Psychotic
         Disorder (310)

.11   With Delusions[I]

.12   With Hallucinations[I]

292.84   Opioid-Induced Mood
         Disorder[I] (370)

292.89   Opioid-Induced Sexual
         Dysfunction[I] (519)

292.89   Opioid-Induced Sleep
         Disorder[I,W] (601)

292.9   Opioid-Related Disorder NOS (255)

PHENCYCLIDINE (OR PHENCYCLIDINE-LIKE)– RELATED DISORDERS (255)
Phencyclidine Use Disorders

304.60   Phencyclidine Dependence[a] (256)

305.90   Phencyclidine Abuse (257)

Phencyclidine-Induced Disorders

292.89   Phencyclidine Intoxication (257)
         Specify if: With Perceptual
         Disturbances

292.81   Phencyclidine Intoxication
         Delirium (129)

292.xx   Phencyclidine-Induced Psychotic
         Disorder (310)

.11   With Delusions[I]

.12   With Hallucinations[I]

292.84   Phencyclidine-Induced Mood
         Disorder[I] (370)

292.89   Phencyclidine-Induced Anxiety
         Disorder[I] (439)

292.9   Phencyclidine-Related Disorder NOS
         (261)

SEDATIVE-, HYPNOTIC-, OR ANXIOLYTIC-RELATED DISORDERS (261)
Sedative, Hypnotic, or Anxiolytic Use Disorders

304.10   Sedative, Hypnotic, or Anxiolytic
         Dependence[a] (262)

305.40   Sedative, Hypnotic, or Anxiolytic
         Abuse (263)

Sedative-, Hypnotic-, or Anxiolytic-Induced Disorders

292.89   Sedative, Hypnotic, or Anxiolytic
         Intoxication (263)

292.0   Sedative, Hypnotic, or Anxiolytic
         Withdrawal (264)
         Specify if: With Perceptual
         Disturbances

292.81   Sedative, Hypnotic, or Anxiolytic
         Intoxication Delirium (129)

292.81   Sedative, Hypnotic, or Anxiolytic
         Withdrawal Delirium (129)

292.82   Sedative-, Hypnotic-, or
         Anxiolytic-Induced Persisting
         Dementia (152)

292.83   Sedative-, Hypnotic-, or
         Anxiolytic-Induced Persisting
         Amnestic Disorder (161)

292.xx   Sedative-, Hypnotic-, or
         Anxiolytic-Induced Psychotic
         Disorder (310)

.11   With Delusions[I,W]

.12   With Hallucinations[I,W]

292.84   Sedative-, Hypnotic-, or
         Anxiolytic-Induced Mood
         Disorder[I,W] (370)

292.89   Sedative-, Hypnotic-, or
         Anxiolytic-Induced Anxiety
         Disorder[W] (439)

292.89   Sedative-, Hypnotic-, or
         Anxiolytic-Induced Sexual
         Dysfunction[I] (519)

292.89   Sedative-, Hypnotic-, or
         Anxiolytic-Induced Sleep
         Disorder[I,W] (601)

292.9   Sedative-, Hypnotic-, or
         Anxiolytic-Related
         Disorder NOS (269)

POLYSUBSTANCE-RELATED DISORDER
304.80   Polysubstance Dependence[a] (270)

OTHER (OR UNKNOWN) SUBSTANCE–RELATED DISORDERS (270)
Other (or Unknown) Substance Use Disorders

304.90   Other (or Unknown) Substance
         Dependence[a] (176)

305.90   Other (or Unknown) Substance
         Abuse (182)

Mood Disorders (317)

Code current state of Major Depressive Disorder or Bipolar I Disorder in fifth digit:

1 = Mild
2 = Moderate
3 = Severe Without Psychotic Features
4 = Severe With Psychotic Features
    Specify: Mood-Congruent Psychotic Features/Mood-Incongruent Psychotic Features
5 = In Partial Remission
6 = In Full Remission
0 = Unspecified

The following specifiers apply (for current or most recent episode) to Mood Disorders as noted.

[a]Severity/Psychotic/Remission Specifiers/[b]Chronic/[c]With Catatonic Features/[d]With Melancholic Features/[e]With Atypical Features/[f]With Postpartum Onset

The following specifiers apply to Mood Disorders as noted:

[g]With or Without Full Interepisode Recovery/[h]With Seasonal Pattern/[i]With Rapid Cycling

DEPRESSIVE DISORDERS

296.xx Major Depressive Disorder, (339)
    .2x   Single Episode[a,b,c,d,e,f]
    .3x   Recurrent[a,b,c,d,e,f,g,h]
300.4   Dysthymic Disorder (345)
    Specify if: Early Onset/Late Onset
    Specify: With Atypical Features
311   Depressive Disorder NOS (350)

BIPOLAR DISORDERS

296.xx Bipolar I Disorder, (350)
    .0x   Single Manic Episode[a,c,f]
    Specify if: Mixed
    .40   Most Recent Episode Hypomanic[g,h,i]
    .4x   Most Recent Episode Manic[a,c,f,g,h,i]
    .6x   Most Recent Episode Mixed[a,c,f,g,h,i]
    .5x   Most Recent Episode Depressed[a,b,c,d,e,f,g,h,i]
    .7   Most Recent Episode Unspecified[g,h,i]
296.89 Bipolar II Disorder[a,b,c,d,e,f,g,h,i] (359)
    Specify (current or most recent episode):
    Hypomanic/Depressed

301.13 Cyclothymic Disorder (363)
296.80 Bipolar Disorder NOS (366)

293.83 Mood Disorder Due to . . . *[Indicate the General Medical Condition]* (366)
    Specify type: With Depressive Features/With Major Depressive–Like Episode/With Manic Features/With Mixed Features
——.—   Substance-Induced Mood Disorder *(refer to Substance-Related Disorders for substance-specific codes)* (370)
    Specify type: With Depressive Features/With Manic Features/With Mixed Features
    Specify if: With Onset During Intoxication/With Onset During Withdrawal

296.90 Mood Disorder NOS (375)

Anxiety Disorders (393)

300.01 Panic Disorder Without Agoraphobia (397)
300.21 Panic Disorder With Agoraphobia (397)
300.22 Agoraphobia Without History of Panic Disorder (403)
300.29 Specific Phobia (405)
    Specify type: Animal Type/Natural Environment Type/Blood-Injection-Injury Type/Situational Type/Other Type
300.23 Social Phobia (411)
    Specify if: Generalized
300.3   Obsessive-Compulsive Disorder (417)
    Specify if: With Poor Insight
309.81 Posttraumatic Stress Disorder (424)
    Specify if: Acute/Chronic
    Specify if: With Delayed Onset
308.3   Acute Stress Disorder (429)
300.02 Generalized Anxiety Disorder (432)
293.84 Anxiety Disorder Due to . . . *[Indicate the General Medical Condition]* (436)
    Specify if: With Generalized Anxiety/With Panic Attacks/With Obsessive-Compulsive Symptoms

——.— Substance-Induced Anxiety Disorder
*(refer to Substance-Related
Disorders for substance-specific
codes)* (439)
Specify if: With Generalized
Anxiety/With Panic Attacks/With
Obsessive-Compulsive
Symptoms/With Phobic
Symptoms
Specify if: With Onset During
Intoxication/With Onset During
Withdrawal

300.00 Anxiety Disorder NOS (444)

Somatoform Disorders (445)

300.81 Somatization Disorder (446)
300.82 Undifferentiated Somatoform
Disorder (450)
300.11 Conversion Disorder (452)
Specify type: With Motor
Symptom or Deficit/With
Sensory Symptom or
Deficit/With Seizures or
Convulsions/With Mixed
Presentation
307.xx Pain Disorder (458)
.80 Associated With
Psychological Factors
.89 Associated With Both
Psychological Factors and a
General Medical Condition
Specify if: Acute/Chronic
300.7 Hypochondriasis (462)
Specify if: With Poor Insight
300.7 Body Dysmorphic Disorder (466)
300.82 Somatoform Disorder NOS (468)

Factitious Disorders (471)

300.xx Factitious Disorder (471)
.16 With Predominantly
Psychological Signs and
Symptoms
.19 With Predominantly Physical
Signs and Symptoms
.19 With Combined Psychological
and Physical Signs and
Symptoms
300.19 Factitious Disorder NOS (475)

Dissociative Disorders (477)

300.12 Dissociative Amnesia (478)
300.13 Dissociative Fugue (481)
300.14 Dissociative Identity Disorder (484)
300.6 Depersonalization Disorder (488)
300.15 Dissociative Disorder NOS (490)

Sexual and Gender Identity Disorders (493)

SEXUAL DYSFUNCTIONS (493)
*The following specifiers apply to all
primary Sexual Dysfunctions:*
Lifelong Type/Acquired Type
Generalized Type/Situational Type
Due to Psychological Factors/Due to
Combined Factors

Sexual Desire Disorders
302.71 Hypoactive Sexual Desire Disorder
(496)
302.79 Sexual Aversion Disorder (499)

Sexual Arousal Disorders
302.72 Female Sexual Arousal
Disorder (500)
302.72 Male Erectile Disorder (502)

Orgasmic Disorders
302.73 Female Orgasmic Disorder (505)
302.74 Male Orgasmic Disorder (507)
302.75 Premature Ejaculation (509)

Sexual Pain Disorders
302.76 Dyspareunia (Not Due to a General
Medical Condition) (511)
306.51 Vaginismus (Not Due to a General
Medical Condition) (513)

**Sexual Dysfunction Due to a
General Medical Condition** (515)
625.8 Female Hypoactive Sexual
Desire Disorder Due to . . .
*[Indicate the General Medical
Condition]* (515)
608.89 Male Hypoactive Sexual
Desire Disorder Due to . . .
*[Indicate the General Medical
Condition]* (515)

607.84 Male Erectile Disorder Due to . . .
        *[Indicate the General Medical
        Condition]* (515)
625.0   Female Dyspareunia Due to . . .
        *[Indicate the General Medical
        Condition]* (515)
608.89 Male Dyspareunia Due to . . .
        *[Indicate the General Medical
        Condition]* (515)
625.8   Other Female Sexual Dysfunction
        Due to . . . *[Indicate the General
        Medical Condition]* (515)
608.89 Other Male Sexual Dysfunction
        Due to . . . *[Indicate the General
        Medical Condition]* (515)
——.–   Substance-Induced Sexual
        Dysfunction *(refer to Substance-
        Related Disorders for substance-
        specific codes)* (519)
        Specify if: With Impaired
        Desire/With Impaired
        Arousal/With Impaired
        Orgasm/With Sexual Pain
        Specify if: With Onset During
        Intoxication

302.70 Sexual Dysfunction NOS (522)

PARAPHILIAS (522)
302.4   Exhibitionism (525)
302.81 Fetishism (526)
302.89 Frotteurism (527)
302.2   Pedophilia (527)
        Specify if: Sexually Attracted to
        Males/Sexually Attracted to
        Females/Sexually Attracted to
        Both
        Specify if: Limited to Incest
        Specify type: Exclusive Type/
        Nonexclusive Type
302.83 Sexual Masochism (529)
302.84 Sexual Sadism (530)
302.3   Transvestic Fetishism (530)
        Specify if: With Gender
        Dysphoria
302.82 Voyeurism (532)
302.9   Paraphilia NOS (532)

GENDER IDENTITY DISORDERS (532)
302.xx Gender Identity Disorder (532)
    .6   in Children
    .85   in Adolescents or Adults
        Specify if: Sexually Attracted to
        Males/Sexually Attracted to
        Females/Sexually Attracted to
        Both/Sexually Attracted to
        Neither
302.6   Gender Identity Disorder
        NOS (538)

302.9   Sexual Disorder NOS (538)

Eating Disorders (539)

307.1   Anorexia Nervosa (539)
        Specify type: Restricting Type;
        Binge-Eating/Purging Type
307.51 Bulimia Nervosa (545)
        Specify type: Purging Type/
        Nonpurging Type
307.50 Eating Disorder NOS (550)

Sleep Disorders (551)

PRIMARY SLEEP DISORDERS (553)
Dyssomnias (553)
307.42 Primary Insomnia (553)
307.44 Primary Hypersomnia (557)
        Specify if: Recurrent
347   Narcolepsy (562)
780.59 Breathing-Related Sleep
        Disorder (567)
307.45 Circadian Rhythm Sleep
        Disorder (573)
        Specify type: Delayed Sleep
        Phase Type/Jet Lag Type/Shift
        Work Type/Unspecified Type
307.47 Dyssomnia NOS (579)

Parasomnias (579)
307.47 Nightmare Disorder (580)
307.46 Sleep Terror Disorder (583)
307.46 Sleepwalking Disorder (587)
307.47 Parasomnia NOS (592)

SLEEP DISORDERS RELATED TO ANOTHER MENTAL DISORDER (592)

307.42 Insomnia Related to . . .
        [Indicate the Axis I or Axis II Disorder] (592)
307.44 Hypersomnia Related to . . .
        [Indicate the Axis I or Axis II Disorder] (592)

OTHER SLEEP DISORDERS

780.xx Sleep Disorder Due to . . . *[Indicate the General Medical Condition]* (597)
   .52   Insomnia Type
   .54   Hypersomnia Type
   .59   Parasomnia Type
   .59   Mixed Type
——.–   Substance-Induced Sleep Disorder *(refer to Substance-Related Disorders for substance-specific codes)* (601)
        Specify type: Insomnia Type/ Hypersomnia Type/Parasomnia Type/Mixed Type
        Specify if: With Onset During Intoxication/With Onset During Withdrawal

Impulse-Control Disorders Not Elsewhere Classified (609)

312.34 Intermittent Explosive Disorder (609)
312.32 Kleptomania (612)
312.33 Pyromania (614)
312.31 Pathological Gambling (615)
312.39 Trichotillomania (618)
312.30 Impulse-Control Disorder NOS (621)

Adjustment Disorders (623)

309.xx Adjustment Disorder (623)
   .0   With Depressed Mood
   .24   With Anxiety
   .28   With Mixed Anxiety and Depressed Mood
   .3   With Disturbance of Conduct
   .4   With Mixed Disturbance of Emotions and Conduct
   .9   Unspecified
        Specify if: Acute/Chronic

Personality Disorders (629)

Note: *These are coded on Axis II.*
301.0   Paranoid Personality Disorder (634)
301.20 Schizoid Personality Disorder (638)
301.22 Schizotypal Personality Disorder (641)
301.7   Antisocial Personality Disorder (645)
301.83 Borderline Personality Disorder (650)
301.50 Histrionic Personality Disorder (655)
301.81 Narcissistic Personality Disorder (658)
301.82 Avoidant Personality Disorder (662)
301.6   Dependent Personality Disorder (665)
301.4   Obsessive-Compulsive Personality Disorder (669)
301.9   Personality Disorder NOS (673)

Other Conditions That May Be a Focus of Clinical Attention (675)

PSYCHOLOGICAL FACTORS AFFECTING MEDICAL CONDITION (675)

316   . . . *[Specified Psychological Factor]* Affecting . . . *[Indicate the General Medical Condition]* (675) *Choose name based on nature of factors:*
         Mental Disorder Affecting Medical Condition
         Psychological Symptoms Affecting Medical Condition
         Personality Traits or Coping Style Affecting Medical Condition
         Maladaptive Health Behaviors Affecting Medical Condition
         Stress-Related Physiological Response Affecting Medical Condition
         Other or Unspecified Psychological Factors Affecting Medical Condition

MEDICATION-INDUCED MOVEMENT DISORDERS (678)

332.1   Neuroleptic-Induced Parkinsonism (679)

333.92 Neuroleptic Malignant Syndrome (679)

333.7   Neuroleptic-Induced Acute Dystonia (679)

333.99 Neuroleptic-Induced Acute Akathisia (679)

333.82 Neuroleptic-Induced Tardive Dyskinesia (679)

333.1   Medication-Induced Postural Tremor (680)

333.90 Medication-Induced Movement Disorder NOS (680)

OTHER MEDICATION-INDUCED DISORDER

995.2   Adverse Effects of Medication NOS (680)

RELATIONAL PROBLEMS (680)

V61.9   Relational Problem Related to a Mental Disorder or General Medical Condition (681)

V61.20 Parent-Child Relational Problem (681)

V61.10 Partner Relational Problem (681)

V61.8   Sibling Relational Problem (681)

V62.81 Relational Problem NOS (681)

PROBLEMS RELATED TO ABUSE OR NEGLECT (682)

V61.21 Physical Abuse of Child (682)
(code 995.54 if focus of attention is on victim)

V61.21 Sexual Abuse of Child (682)
(code 995.53 if focus of attention is on victim)

V61.21 Neglect of Child (682)
(code 995.52 if focus of attention is on victim)

——.— Physical Abuse of Adult (682)

V61.12   (if by partner)

V62.83   (if by person other than partner)
(code 995.81 if focus of attention is on victim)

——.— Sexual Abuse of Adult (682)

V61.12   (if by partner)

V62.83   (if by person other than partner)
(code 995.83 if focus of attention is on victim)

ADDITIONAL CONDITIONS THAT MAY BE A FOCUS OF CLINICAL ATTENTION (683)

V15.81 Noncompliance With Treatment (683)

V65.2   Malingering (683)

V71.01 Adult Antisocial Behavior (683)

V71.02 Child or Adolescent Antisocial Behavior (684)

V62.89 Borderline Intellectual Functioning (684)
Note: This is coded on Axis II.

780.9   Age-Related Cognitive Decline (684)

V62.82 Bereavement (684)

V62.3   Academic Problem (685)

V62.2   Occupational Problem (685)

313.82 Identity Problem (685)

V62.89 Religious or Spiritual Problem (685)

V62.4   Acculturation Problem (685)

V62.89 Phase of Life Problem (685)

Additional Codes

300.9   Unspecified Mental Disorder (nonpsychotic) (687)

V71.09 No Diagnosis or Condition on Axis I (687)

799.9   Diagnosis or Condition Deferred on Axis I (687)

V71.09 No Diagnosis on Axis II (687)

799.9   Diagnosis Deferred on Axis II (687)

Multiaxial System

Axis I   Clinical Disorders
Other Conditions That May Be a Focus of Clinical Attention

Axis II Personality Disorders
Mental Retardation

Axis III General Medical Conditions

Axis IV Psychosocial and Environmental Problems

Axis V   Global Assessment of Functioning

Appendix E

Alphabetical Listing of DSM-IV Diagnoses and Codes

Updated to include ICD-9-CM codes effective October 1, 1996

NOS = Not Otherwise Specified.

V62.3	Academic Problem
V62.4	Acculturation Problem
308.3	Acute Stress Disorder
	Adjustment Disorders
309.9	Unspecified
309.24	With Anxiety
309.0	With Depressed Mood
309.3	With Disturbance of Conduct
309.28	With Mixed Anxiety and Depressed Mood
309.4	With Mixed Disturbance of Emotions and Conduct
V71.01	Adult Antisocial Behavior
995.2	Adverse Effects of Medication NOS
780.9	Age-Related Cognitive Decline
300.22	Agoraphobia Without History of Panic Disorder
	Alcohol
305.00	Abuse
303.90	Dependence
291.89	-Induced Anxiety Disorder
291.89	-Induced Mood Disorder
291.1	-Induced Persisting Amnestic Disorder
291.2	-Induced Persisting Dementia
	-Induced Psychotic Disorder
291.5	With Delusions
291.3	With Hallucinations
291.89	-Induced Sexual Dysfunction
291.89	-Induced Sleep Disorder
303.00	Intoxication
291.0	Intoxication Delirium
291.9	-Related Disorder NOS
291.81	Withdrawal
291.0	Withdrawal Delirium

33

294.0	Amnestic Disorder Due to . . . *[Indicate the General Medical Condition]*
294.8	Amnestic Disorder NOS
	Amphetamine (or Amphetamine-Like)
305.70	Abuse
304.40	Dependence
292.89	-Induced Anxiety Disorder
292.84	-Induced Mood Disorder
	-Induced Psychotic Disorder
292.11	With Delusions
292.12	With Hallucinations
292.89	-Induced Sexual Dysfunction
292.89	-Induced Sleep Disorder
292.89	Intoxication
292.81	Intoxication Delirium
292.9	-Related Disorder NOS
292.0	Withdrawal
307.1	Anorexia Nervosa
301.7	Antisocial Personality Disorder
293.84	Anxiety Disorder Due to . . . *[Indicate the General Medical Condition]*
300.00	Anxiety Disorder NOS
299.80	Asperger's Disorder
	Attention-Deficit/Hyperactivity Disorder
314.01	Combined Type
314.01	Predominantly Hyperactive-Impulsive Type
314.00	Predominantly Inattentive Type
314.9	Attention-Deficit/Hyperactivity Disorder NOS
299.00	Autistic Disorder
301.82	Avoidant Personality Disorder
V62.82	Bereavement
296.80	Bipolar Disorder NOS
	Bipolar I Disorder, Most Recent Episode Depressed
296.56	In Full Remission
296.55	In Partial Remission
296.51	Mild
296.52	Moderate
296.53	Severe Without Psychotic Features
296.54	Severe With Psychotic Features
296.50	Unspecified
296.40	Bipolar I Disorder, Most Recent Episode Hypomanic
	Bipolar I Disorder, Most Recent Episode Manic
296.46	In Full Remission
296.45	In Partial Remission
296.41	Mild
296.42	Moderate
296.43	Severe Without Psychotic Features
296.44	Severe With Psychotic Features
296.40	Unspecified
	Bipolar I Disorder, Most Recent Episode Mixed
296.66	In Full Remission
296.65	In Partial Remission
296.61	Mild

Bipolar I Disorder, Most Recent Episode Mixed *(continued)*

296.62	Moderate
296.63	Severe Without Psychotic Features
296.64	Severe With Psychotic Features
296.60	Unspecified
296.7	Bipolar I Disorder, Most Recent Episode Unspecified
	Bipolar I Disorder, Single Manic Episode
296.06	In Full Remission
296.05	In Partial Remission
296.01	Mild
296.02	Moderate
296.03	Severe Without Psychotic Features
296.04	Severe With Psychotic Features
296.00	Unspecified
296.89	Bipolar II Disorder
300.7	Body Dysmorphic Disorder
V62.89	Borderline Intellectual Functioning
301.83	Borderline Personality Disorder
780.59	Breathing-Related Sleep Disorder
298.8	Brief Psychotic Disorder
307.51	Bulimia Nervosa
	Caffeine
292.89	-Induced Anxiety Disorder
292.89	-Induced Sleep Disorder
305.90	Intoxication
292.9	-Related Disorder NOS
	Cannabis
305.20	Abuse
304.30	Dependence
292.89	-Induced Anxiety Disorder
	-Induced Psychotic Disorder
292.11	With Delusions
292.12	With Hallucinations
292.89	Intoxication
292.81	Intoxication Delirium
292.9	-Related Disorder NOS
293.89	Catatonic Disorder Due to . . . *[Indicate the General Medical Condition]*
299.10	Childhood Disintegrative Disorder
V71.02	Child or Adolescent Antisocial Behavior
307.22	Chronic Motor or Vocal Tic Disorder
307.45	Circadian Rhythm Sleep Disorder
	Cocaine
305.60	Abuse
304.20	Dependence
292.89	-Induced Anxiety Disorder
292.84	-Induced Mood Disorder
	-Induced Psychotic Disorder
292.11	With Delusions
292.12	With Hallucinations
292.89	-Induced Sexual Dysfunction
292.89	-Induced Sleep Disorder

	Cocaine *(continued)*
292.89	Intoxication
292.81	Intoxication Delirium
292.9	-Related Disorder NOS
292.0	Withdrawal
294.9	Cognitive Disorder NOS
307.9	Communication Disorder NOS
	Conduct Disorder
312.81	Childhood-Onset Type
312.82	Adolescent-Onset Type
312.89	Unspecified Onset
300.11	Conversion Disorder
301.13	Cyclothymic Disorder
293.0	Delirium Due to . . . *[Indicate the General Medical Condition]*
/80.09	Delirium NOS
297.1	Delusional Disorder
290.10	Dementia Due to Creutzfeldt-Jakob Disease
294.1	Dementia Due to Head Trauma
294.1	Dementia Due to HIV Disease
294.1	Dementia Due to Huntington's Disease
294.1	Dementia Due to Parkinson's Disease
290.10	Dementia Due to Pick's Disease
294.1	Dementia Due to . . . *[Indicate Other General Medical Condition]*
294.8	Dementia NOS
	Dementia of the Alzheimer's Type, With Early Onset
290.10	Uncomplicated
290.11	With Delirium
290.12	With Delusions
290.13	With Depressed Mood
	Dementia of the Alzheimer's Type, With Late Onset
290.0	Uncomplicated
290.3	With Delirium
290.20	With Delusions
290.21	With Depressed Mood
301.6	Dependent Personality Disorder
300.6	Depersonalization Disorder
311	Depressive Disorder NOS
315.4	Developmental Coordination Disorder
799.9	Diagnosis Deferred on Axis II
799.9	Diagnosis or Condition Deferred on Axis I
313.9	Disorder of Infancy, Childhood, or Adolescence NOS
315.2	Disorder of Written Expression
312.9	Disruptive Behavior Disorder NOS
300.12	Dissociative Amnesia
300.15	Dissociative Disorder NOS
300.13	Dissociative Fugue
300.14	Dissociative Identity Disorder
302.76	Dyspareunia (Not Due to a General Medical Condition)
307.47	Dyssomnia NOS
300.4	Dysthymic Disorder
307.50	Eating Disorder NOS

787.6	Encopresis, With Constipation and Overflow Incontinence
307.7	Encopresis, Without Constipation and Overflow Incontinence
307.6	Enuresis (Not Due to a General Medical Condition)
302.4	Exhibitionism
315.31	Expressive Language Disorder
	Factitious Disorder
300.19	With Combined Psychological and Physical Signs and Symptoms
300.19	With Predominantly Physical Signs and Symptoms
300.16	With Predominantly Psychological Signs and Symptoms
300.19	Factitious Disorder NOS
307.59	Feeding Disorder of Infancy or Early Childhood
625.0	Female Dyspareunia Due to . . . *[Indicate the General Medical Condition]*
625.8	Female Hypoactive Sexual Desire Disorder Due to . . . *[Indicate the General Medical Condition]*
302.73	Female Orgasmic Disorder
302.72	Female Sexual Arousal Disorder
302.81	Fetishism
302.89	Frotteurism
	Gender Identity Disorder
302.85	in Adolescents or Adults
302.6	in Children
302.6	Gender Identity Disorder NOS
300.02	Generalized Anxiety Disorder
	Hallucinogen
305.30	Abuse
304.50	Dependence
292.89	-Induced Anxiety Disorder
292.84	-Induced Mood Disorder
	-Induced Psychotic Disorder
292.11	With Delusions
292.12	With Hallucinations
292.89	Intoxication
292.81	Intoxication Delirium
292.89	Persisting Perception Disorder
292.9	-Related Disorder NOS
301.50	Histrionic Personality Disorder
307.44	Hypersomnia related to . . . *[Indicate the Axis I or Axis II Disorder]*
302.71	Hypoactive Sexual Desire Disorder
300.7	Hypochondriasis
313.82	Identity Problem
312.30	Impulse-Control Disorder NOS
	Inhalant
305.90	Abuse
304.60	Dependence
292.89	-Induced Anxiety Disorder
292.84	-Induced Mood Disorder
292.82	-Induced Persisting Dementia
	-Induced Psychotic Disorder
292.11	With Delusions
292.12	With Hallucinations

Inhalant *(continued)*

292.89	Intoxication
292.81	Intoxication Delirium
292.9	-Related Disorder NOS
307.42	Insomnia Related to . . . *[Indicate the Axis I or Axis II Disorder]*
312.34	Intermittent Explosive Disorder
312.32	Kleptomania
315.9	Learning Disorder NOS

Major Depressive Disorder, Recurrent

296.36	In Full Remission
296.35	In Partial Remission
296.31	Mild
296.32	Moderate
296.33	Severe Without Psychotic Features
296.34	Severe With Psychotic Features
296.30	Unspecified

Major Depressive Disorder, Single Episode

296.26	In Full Remission
296.25	In Partial Remission
296.21	Mild
296.22	Moderate
296.23	Severe Without Psychotic Features
296.24	Severe With Psychotic Features
296.20	Unspecified
608.89	Male Dyspareunia Due to . . . *[Indicate the General Medical Condition]*
302.72	Male Erectile Disorder
607.84	Male Erectile Disorder Due to . . . *[Indicate the General Medical Condition]*
608.89	Male Hypoactive Sexual Desire Disorder Due to . . . *[Indicate the General Medical Condition]*
302.74	Male Orgasmic Disorder
V65.2	Malingering
315.1	Mathematics Disorder

Medication-Induced

333.90	Movement Disorder NOS
333.1	Postural Tremor
293.9	Mental Disorder NOS Due to . . . *[Indicate the General Medical Condition]*
319	Mental Retardation, Severity Unspecified
317	Mild Mental Retardation
315.32	Mixed Receptive-Expressive Language Disorder
318.0	Moderate Mental Retardation
293.83	Mood Disorder Due to . . . *[Indicate the General Medical Condition]*
296.90	Mood Disorder NOS
301.81	Narcissistic Personality Disorder
347	Narcolepsy
V61.21	Neglect of Child
995.52	Neglect of Child *(if focus of attention is on victim)*

Neuroleptic-Induced

333.99	Acute Akathisia
333.7	Acute Dystonia
332.1	Parkinsonism
333.82	Tardive Dyskinesia

	Panic Disorder
300.21	With Agoraphobia
300.01	Without Agoraphobia
301.0	Paranoid Personality Disorder
302.9	Paraphilia NOS
307.47	Parasomnia NOS
V61.20	Parent-Child Relational Problem
V61.10	Partner Relational Problem
312.31	Pathological Gambling
302.2	Pedophilia
310.1	Personality Change Due to . . . *[Indicate the General Medical Condition]*
301.9	Personality Disorder NOS
299.80	Pervasive Developmental Disorder NOS
V62.89	Phase of Life Problem
	Phencyclidine (or Phencyclidine-Like)
305.90	Abuse
304.60	Dependence
292.89	–Induced Anxiety Disorder
292.84	–Induced Mood Disorder
	–Induced Psychotic Disorder
292.11	With Delusions
292.12	With Hallucinations
292.89	Intoxication
292.81	Intoxication Delirium
292.9	–Related Disorder NOS
315.39	Phonological Disorder
V61.12	Physical Abuse of Adult (if by partner)
V62.83	Physical Abuse of Adult (if by person other than partner)
995.81	Physical Abuse of Adult *(if focus of attention is on victim)*
V61.21	Physical Abuse of Child
995.54	Physical Abuse of Child *(if focus of attention is on victim)*
307.52	Pica
304.80	Polysubstance Dependence
309.81	Posttraumatic Stress Disorder
302.75	Premature Ejaculation
307.44	Primary Hypersomnia
307.42	Primary Insomnia
318.2	Profound Mental Retardation
316	Psychological Factors Affecting Medical Condition
	Psychotic Disorder Due to . . . *[Indicate the General Medical Condition]*
293.81	With Delusions
293.82	With Hallucinations
298.9	Psychotic Disorder NOS
312.33	Pyromania
313.89	Reactive Attachment Disorder of Infancy or Early Childhood
315.00	Reading Disorder
V62.81	Relational Problem NOS
V61.9	Relational Problem Related to a Mental Disorder or General Medical Condition
V62.89	Religious or Spiritual Problem
299.80	Rett's Disorder
307.53	Rumination Disorder

295.70	Schizoaffective Disorder
301.20	Schizoid Personality Disorder
	Schizophrenia
295.20	Catatonic Type
295.10	Disorganized Type
295.30	Paranoid Type
295.60	Residual Type
295.90	Undifferentiated Type
295.40	Schizophreniform Disorder
301.22	Schizotypal Personality Disorder
	Sedative, Hypnotic, or Anxiolytic
305.40	Abuse
304.10	Dependence
292.89	-Induced Anxiety Disorder
292.84	-Induced Mood Disorder
292.83	-Induced Persisting Amnestic Disorder
292.82	-Induced Persisting Dementia
	-Induced Psychotic Disorder
292.11	With Delusions
292.12	With Hallucinations
292.89	-Induced Sexual Dysfunction
292.89	-Induced Sleep Disorder
292.89	Intoxication
292.81	Intoxication Delirium
292.9	-Related Disorder NOS
292.0	Withdrawal
292.81	Withdrawal Delirium
313.23	Selective Mutism
309.21	Separation Anxiety Disorder
318.1	Severe Mental Retardation
V61.12	Sexual Abuse of Adult (if by partner)
V62.83	Sexual Abuse of Adult (if by person other than partner)
995.83	Sexual Abuse of Adult *(if focus of attention is on victim)*
V61.21	Sexual Abuse of Child
995.53	Sexual Abuse of Child *(if focus of attention is on victim)*
302.79	Sexual Aversion Disorder
302.9	Sexual Disorder NOS
302.70	Sexual Dysfunction NOS
302.83	Sexual Masochism
302.84	Sexual Sadism
297.3	Shared Psychotic Disorder
V61.8	Sibling Relational Problem
	Sleep Disorder Due to . . . *[Indicate the General Medical Condition]*
780.54	Hypersomnia Type
780.52	Insomnia Type
780.59	Mixed Type
780.59	Parasomnia Type
307.46	Sleep Terror Disorder
307.46	Sleepwalking Disorder
300.23	Social Phobia
300.81	Somatization Disorder

300.82	Somatoform Disorder NOS
300.29	Specific Phobia
307.3	Stereotypic Movement Disorder
307.0	Stuttering
307.20	Tic Disorder NOS
307.23	Tourette's Disorder
307.21	Transient Tic Disorder
302.3	Transvestic Fetishism
312.39	Trichotillomania
300.82	Undifferentiated Somatoform Disorder
300.9	Unspecified Mental Disorder (nonpsychotic)
306.51	Vaginismus (Not Due to a General Medical Condition)
	Vascular Dementia
290.40	Uncomplicated
290.41	With Delirium
290.42	With Delusions
290.43	With Depressed Mood
302.82	Voyeurism

Appendix F

Numerical Listing of DSM-IV Diagnoses and Codes

Updated to include ICD-9-CM codes effective October 1, 1996

To maintain compatibility with ICD-9-CM, some DSM-IV diagnoses share the same code numbers. These are indicated in this list by brackets.

NOS = Not Otherwise Specified.

290.0	Dementia of the Alzheimer's Type, With Late Onset, Uncomplicated
290.10	Dementia Due to Creutzfeldt-Jakob Disease
290.10	Dementia Due to Pick's Disease
290.10	Dementia of the Alzheimer's Type, With Early Onset, Uncomplicated
290.11	Dementia of the Alzheimer's Type, With Early Onset, With Delirium
290.12	Dementia of the Alzheimer's Type, With Early Onset, With Delusions
290.13	Dementia of the Alzheimer's Type, With Early Onset, With Depressed Mood
290.20	Dementia of the Alzheimer's Type, With Late Onset, With Delusions
290.21	Dementia of the Alzheimer's Type, With Late Onset, With Depressed Mood
290.3	Dementia of the Alzheimer's Type, With Late Onset, With Delirium
290.40	Vascular Dementia, Uncomplicated
290.41	Vascular Dementia, With Delirium
290.42	Vascular Dementia, With Delusions
290.43	Vascular Dementia, With Depressed Mood
291.0	Alcohol Intoxication Delirium
291.0	Alcohol Withdrawal Delirium
291.1	Alcohol-Induced Persisting Amnestic Disorder
291.2	Alcohol-Induced Persisting Dementia
291.3	Alcohol-Induced Psychotic Disorder, With Hallucinations
291.5	Alcohol-Induced Psychotic Disorder, With Delusions
291.81	Alcohol Withdrawal
291.89	Alcohol-Induced Anxiety Disorder
291.89	Alcohol-Induced Mood Disorder
291.89	Alcohol-Induced Sexual Dysfunction
291.89	Alcohol-Induced Sleep Disorder

291.9   Alcohol-Related Disorder NOS
292.0   Amphetamine Withdrawal
292.0   Cocaine Withdrawal
292.0   Nicotine Withdrawal
292.0   Opioid Withdrawal
292.0   Other (or Unknown) Substance Withdrawal
292.0   Sedative, Hypnotic, or Anxiolytic Withdrawal
292.11   Amphetamine-Induced Psychotic Disorder, With Delusions
292.11   Cannabis-Induced Psychotic Disorder, With Delusions
292.11   Cocaine-Induced Psychotic Disorder, With Delusions
292.11   Hallucinogen-Induced Psychotic Disorder, With Delusions
292.11   Inhalant-Induced Psychotic Disorder, With Delusions
292.11   Opioid-Induced Psychotic Disorder, With Delusions
292.11   Other (or Unknown) Substance–Induced Psychotic Disorder,
          With Delusions
292.11   Phencyclidine-Induced Psychotic Disorder, With Delusions
292.11   Sedative-, Hypnotic-, or Anxiolytic-Induced Psychotic Disorder, With Delusions
292.12   Amphetamine-Induced Psychotic Disorder, With Hallucinations
292.12   Cannabis-Induced Psychotic Disorder, With Hallucinations
292.12   Cocaine-Induced Psychotic Disorder, With Hallucinations
292.12   Hallucinogen-Induced Psychotic Disorder, With Hallucinations
292.12   Inhalant-Induced Psychotic Disorder, With Hallucinations
292.12   Opioid-Induced Psychotic Disorder, With Hallucinations
292.12   Other (or Unknown) Substance–Induced Psychotic Disorder,
          With Hallucinations
292.12   Phencyclidine-Induced Psychotic Disorder, With Hallucinations
292.12   Sedative-, Hypnotic-, or Anxiolytic-Induced Psychotic Disorder,
          With Hallucinations
292.81   Amphetamine Intoxication Delirium
292.81   Cannabis Intoxication Delirium
292.81   Cocaine Intoxication Delirium
292.81   Hallucinogen Intoxication Delirium
292.81   Inhalant Intoxication Delirium
292.81   Opioid Intoxication Delirium
292.81   Other (or Unknown) Substance–Induced Delirium
292.81   Phencyclidine Intoxication Delirium
292.81   Sedative, Hypnotic, or Anxiolytic Intoxication Delirium
292.81   Sedative, Hypnotic, or Anxiolytic Withdrawal Delirium
292.82   Inhalant-Induced Persisting Dementia
292.82   Other (or Unknown) Substance–Induced Persisting Dementia
292.82   Sedative-, Hypnotic-, or Anxiolytic-Induced Persisting Dementia
292.83   Other (or Unknown) Substance–Induced Persisting Amnestic Disorder
292.83   Sedative-, Hypnotic-, or Anxiolytic-Induced Persisting Amnestic Disorder
292.84   Amphetamine-Induced Mood Disorder
292.84   Cocaine-Induced Mood Disorder
292.84   Hallucinogen-Induced Mood Disorder
292.84   Inhalant-Induced Mood Disorder
292.84   Opioid-Induced Mood Disorder
292.84   Other (or Unknown) Substance–Induced Mood Disorder
292.84   Phencyclidine-Induced Mood Disorder
292.84   Sedative-, Hypnotic-, or Anxiolytic-Induced Mood Disorder

292.89   Amphetamine-Induced Anxiety Disorder
292.89   Amphetamine-Induced Sexual Dysfunction
292.89   Amphetamine-Induced Sleep Disorder
292.89   Amphetamine Intoxication
292.89   Caffeine-Induced Anxiety Disorder
292.89   Caffeine-Induced Sleep Disorder
292.89   Cannabis-Induced Anxiety Disorder
292.89   Cannabis Intoxication
292.89   Cocaine-Induced Anxiety Disorder
292.89   Cocaine-Induced Sexual Dysfunction
292.89   Cocaine-Induced Sleep Disorder
292.89   Cocaine Intoxication
292.89   Hallucinogen-Induced Anxiety Disorder
292.89   Hallucinogen Intoxication
292.89   Hallucinogen Persisting Perception Disorder
292.89   Inhalant-Induced Anxiety Disorder
292.89   Inhalant Intoxication
292.89   Opioid-Induced Sleep Disorder
292.89   Opioid-Induced Sexual Dysfunction
292.89   Opioid Intoxication
292.89   Other (or Unknown) Substance–Induced Anxiety Disorder
292.89   Other (or Unknown) Substance–Induced Sexual Dysfunction
292.89   Other (or Unknown) Substance–Induced Sleep Disorder
292.89   Other (or Unknown) Substance Intoxication
292.89   Phencyclidine-Induced Anxiety Disorder
292.89   Phencyclidine Intoxication
292.89   Sedative-, Hypnotic-, or Anxiolytic-Induced Anxiety Disorder
292.89   Sedative-, Hypnotic-, or Anxiolytic-Induced Sexual Dysfunction
292.89   Sedative-, Hypnotic-, or Anxiolytic-Induced Sleep Disorder
292.89   Sedative, Hypnotic, or Anxiolytic Intoxication
292.9   Amphetamine-Related Disorder NOS
292.9   Caffeine-Related Disorder NOS
292.9   Cannabis-Related Disorder NOS
292.9   Cocaine-Related Disorder NOS
292.9   Hallucinogen-Related Disorder NOS
292.9   Inhalant-Related Disorder NOS
292.9   Nicotine-Related Disorder NOS
292.9   Opioid-Related Disorder NOS
292.9   Other (or Unknown) Substance–Related Disorder NOS
292.9   Phencyclidine-Related Disorder NOS
292.9   Sedative-, Hypnotic-, or Anxiolytic-Related Disorder NOS
293.0   Delirium Due to . . . *[Indicate the General Medical Condition]*
293.81   Psychotic Disorder Due to . . . *[Indicate the General Medical Condition]*, With Delusions
293.82   Psychotic Disorder Due to . . . *[Indicate the General Medical Condition]*, With Hallucinations
293.83   Mood Disorder Due to . . . *[Indicate the General Medical Condition]*
293.84   Anxiety Disorder Due to . . . *[Indicate the General Medical Condition]*
293.89   Catatonic Disorder Due to . . . *[Indicate the General Medical Condition]*
293.9   Mental Disorder NOS Due to . . . *[Indicate the General Medical Condition]*
294.0   Amnestic Disorder Due to . . . *[Indicate the General Medical Condition]*

294.1	Dementia Due to . . . *[Indicate the General Medical Condition]*
294.8	Amnestic Disorder NOS
294.8	Dementia NOS
294.9	Cognitive Disorder NOS
295.10	Schizophrenia, Disorganized Type
295.20	Schizophrenia, Catatonic Type
295.30	Schizophrenia, Paranoid Type
295.40	Schizophreniform Disorder
295.60	Schizophrenia, Residual Type
295.70	Schizoaffective Disorder
295.90	Schizophrenia, Undifferentiated Type
296.00	Bipolar I Disorder, Single Manic Episode, Unspecified
296.01	Bipolar I Disorder, Single Manic Episode, Mild
296.02	Bipolar I Disorder, Single Manic Episode, Moderate
296.03	Bipolar I Disorder, Single Manic Episode, Severe Without Psychotic Features
296.04	Bipolar I Disorder, Single Manic Episode, Severe With Psychotic Features
296.05	Bipolar I Disorder, Single Manic Episode, In Partial Remission
296.06	Bipolar I Disorder, Single Manic Episode, In Full Remission
296.20	Major Depressive Disorder, Single Episode, Unspecified
296.21	Major Depressive Disorder, Single Episode, Mild
296.22	Major Depressive Disorder, Single Episode, Moderate
296.23	Major Depressive Disorder, Single Episode, Severe Without Psychotic Features
296.24	Major Depressive Disorder, Single Episode, Severe With Psychotic Features
296.25	Major Depressive Disorder, Single Episode, In Partial Remission
296.26	Major Depressive Disorder, Single Episode, In Full Remission
296.30	Major Depressive Disorder, Recurrent, Unspecified
296.31	Major Depressive Disorder, Recurrent, Mild
296.32	Major Depressive Disorder, Recurrent, Moderate
296.33	Major Depressive Disorder, Recurrent, Severe Without Psychotic Features
296.34	Major Depressive Disorder, Recurrent, Severe With Psychotic Features
296.35	Major Depressive Disorder, Recurrent, In Partial Remission
296.36	Major Depressive Disorder, Recurrent, In Full Remission
296.40	Bipolar I Disorder, Most Recent Episode Hypomanic
296.40	Bipolar I Disorder, Most Recent Episode Manic, Unspecified
296.41	Bipolar I Disorder, Most Recent Episode Manic, Mild
296.42	Bipolar I Disorder, Most Recent Episode Manic, Moderate
296.43	Bipolar I Disorder, Most Recent Episode Manic, Severe Without Psychotic Features
296.44	Bipolar I Disorder, Most Recent Episode Manic, Severe With Psychotic Features
296.45	Bipolar I Disorder, Most Recent Episode Manic, In Partial Remission
296.46	Bipolar I Disorder, Most Recent Episode Manic, In Full Remission
296.50	Bipolar I Disorder, Most Recent Episode Depressed, Unspecified
296.51	Bipolar I Disorder, Most Recent Episode Depressed, Mild
296.52	Bipolar I Disorder, Most Recent Episode Depressed, Moderate
296.53	Bipolar I Disorder, Most Recent Episode Depressed, Severe Without Psychotic Features
296.54	Bipolar I Disorder, Most Recent Episode Depressed, Severe With Psychotic Features

296.55	Bipolar I Disorder, Most Recent Episode Depressed, In Partial Remission
296.56	Bipolar I Disorder, Most Recent Episode Depressed, In Full Remission
296.60	Bipolar I Disorder, Most Recent Episode Mixed, Unspecified
296.61	Bipolar I Disorder, Most Recent Episode Mixed, Mild
296.62	Bipolar I Disorder, Most Recent Episode Mixed, Moderate
296.63	Bipolar I Disorder, Most Recent Episode Mixed, Severe Without Psychotic Features
296.64	Bipolar I Disorder, Most Recent Episode Mixed, Severe With Psychotic Features
296.65	Bipolar I Disorder, Most Recent Episode Mixed, In Partial Remission
296.66	Bipolar I Disorder, Most Recent Episode Mixed, In Full Remission
296.7	Bipolar I Disorder, Most Recent Episode Unspecified
296.80	Bipolar Disorder NOS
296.89	Bipolar II Disorder
296.90	Mood Disorder NOS
297.1	Delusional Disorder
297.3	Shared Psychotic Disorder
298.8	Brief Psychotic Disorder
298.9	Psychotic Disorder NOS
299.00	Autistic Disorder
299.10	Childhood Disintegrative Disorder
⌈ 299.80	Asperger's Disorder
299.80	Pervasive Developmental Disorder NOS
⌊ 299.80	Rett's Disorder
300.00	Anxiety Disorder NOS
300.01	Panic Disorder Without Agoraphobia
300.02	Generalized Anxiety Disorder
300.11	Conversion Disorder
300.12	Dissociative Amnesia
300.13	Dissociative Fugue
300.14	Dissociative Identity Disorder
300.15	Dissociative Disorder NOS
300.16	Factitious Disorder With Predominantly Psychological Signs and Symptoms
⌈ 300.19	Factitious Disorder NOS
300.19	Factitious Disorder With Combined Psychological and Physical Signs and Symptoms
⌊ 300.19	Factitious Disorder With Predominantly Physical Signs and Symptoms
300.21	Panic Disorder With Agoraphobia
300.22	Agoraphobia Without History of Panic Disorder
300.23	Social Phobia
300.29	Specific Phobia
300.3	Obsessive-Compulsive Disorder
300.4	Dysthymic Disorder
300.6	Depersonalization Disorder
⌈ 300.7	Body Dysmorphic Disorder
⌊ 300.7	Hypochondriasis
300.81	Somatization Disorder
⌈ 300.82	Somatoform Disorder NOS
⌊ 300.82	Undifferentiated Somatoform Disorder
300.9	Unspecified Mental Disorder (nonpsychotic)
301.0	Paranoid Personality Disorder

301.13	Cyclothymic Disorder
301.20	Schizoid Personality Disorder
301.22	Schizotypal Personality Disorder
301.4	Obsessive-Compulsive Personality Disorder
301.50	Histrionic Personality Disorder
301.6	Dependent Personality Disorder
301.7	Antisocial Personality Disorder
301.81	Narcissistic Personality Disorder
301.82	Avoidant Personality Disorder
301.83	Borderline Personality Disorder
301.9	Personality Disorder NOS
302.2	Pedophilia
302.3	Transvestic Fetishism
302.4	Exhibitionism
⌐ 302.6	Gender Identity Disorder in Children
⌐ 302.6	Gender Identity Disorder NOS
302.70	Sexual Dysfunction NOS
302.71	Hypoactive Sexual Desire Disorder
⌐ 302.72	Female Sexual Arousal Disorder
⌐ 302.72	Male Erectile Disorder
302.73	Female Orgasmic Disorder
302.74	Male Orgasmic Disorder
302.75	Premature Ejaculation
302.76	Dyspareunia (Not Due to a General Medical Condition)
302.79	Sexual Aversion Disorder
302.81	Fetishism
302.82	Voyeurism
302.83	Sexual Masochism
302.84	Sexual Sadism
302.85	Gender Identity Disorder in Adolescents or Adults
302.89	Frotteurism
⌐ 302.9	Paraphilia NOS
⌐ 302.9	Sexual Disorder NOS
303.00	Alcohol Intoxication
303.90	Alcohol Dependence
304.00	Opioid Dependence
304.10	Sedative, Hypnotic, or Anxiolytic Dependence
304.20	Cocaine Dependence
304.30	Cannabis Dependence
304.40	Amphetamine Dependence
304.50	Hallucinogen Dependence
⌐ 304.60	Inhalant Dependence
⌐ 304.60	Phencyclidine Dependence
304.80	Polysubstance Dependence
304.90	Other (or Unknown) Substance Dependence
305.00	Alcohol Abuse
305.10	Nicotine Dependence
305.20	Cannabis Abuse
305.30	Hallucinogen Abuse
305.40	Sedative, Hypnotic, or Anxiolytic Abuse
305.50	Opioid Abuse

305.60   Cocaine Abuse
305.70   Amphetamine Abuse
⌐ 305.90   Caffeine Intoxication
| 305.90   Inhalant Abuse
| 305.90   Other (or Unknown) Substance Abuse
└ 305.90   Phencyclidine Abuse
306.51   Vaginismus (Not Due to a General Medical Condition)
307.0   Stuttering
307.1   Anorexia Nervosa
307.20   Tic Disorder NOS
307.21   Transient Tic Disorder
307.22   Chronic Motor or Vocal Tic Disorder
307.23   Tourette's Disorder
307.3   Stereotypic Movement Disorder
⌐ 307.42   Insomnia Related to . . . *[Indicate the Axis I or Axis II Disorder]*
└ 307.42   Primary Insomnia
⌐ 307.44   Hypersomnia Related to . . . *[Indicate the Axis I or Axis II Disorder]*
└ 307.44   Primary Hypersomnia
307.45   Circadian Rhythm Sleep Disorder
⌐ 307.46   Sleep Terror Disorder
└ 307.46   Sleepwalking Disorder
⌐ 307.47   Dyssomnia NOS
| 307.47   Nightmare Disorder
└ 307.47   Parasomnia NOS
307.50   Eating Disorder NOS
307.51   Bulimia Nervosa
307.52   Pica
307.53   Rumination Disorder
307.59   Feeding Disorder of Infancy or Early Childhood
307.6   Enuresis (Not Due to a General Medical Condition)
307.7   Encopresis, Without Constipation and Overflow Incontinence
307.80   Pain Disorder Associated With Psychological Factors
307.89   Pain Disorder Associated With Both Psychological Factors and a
          General Medical Condition
307.9   Communication Disorder NOS
308.3   Acute Stress Disorder
309.0   Adjustment Disorder With Depressed Mood
309.21   Separation Anxiety Disorder
309.24   Adjustment Disorder With Anxiety
309.28   Adjustment Disorder With Mixed Anxiety and Depressed Mood
309.3   Adjustment Disorder With Disturbance of Conduct
309.4   Adjustment Disorder With Mixed Disturbance of Emotions and Conduct
309.81   Posttraumatic Stress Disorder
309.9   Adjustment Disorder Unspecified
310.1   Personality Change Due to . . . *[Indicate the General Medical Condition]*
311   Depressive Disorder NOS
312.30   Impulse-Control Disorder NOS
312.31   Pathological Gambling
312.32   Kleptomania
312.33   Pyromania
312.34   Intermittent Explosive Disorder

312.39	Trichotillomania
312.81	Conduct Disorder, Childhood-Onset Type
312.82	Conduct Disorder, Adolescent-Onset Type
312.89	Conduct Disorder, Unspecified Onset
312.9	Disruptive Behavior Disorder NOS
313.23	Selective Mutism
313.81	Oppositional Defiant Disorder
313.82	Identity Problem
313.89	Reactive Attachment Disorder of Infancy or Early Childhood
313.9	Disorder of Infancy, Childhood, or Adolescence NOS
314.00	Attention-Deficit/Hyperactivity Disorder, Predominantly Inattentive Type
314.01	Attention-Deficit/Hyperactivity Disorder, Combined Type
314.01	Attention-Deficit/Hyperactivity Disorder, Predominantly Hyperactive-Impulsive Type
314.9	Attention-Deficit/Hyperactivity Disorder NOS
315.00	Reading Disorder
315.1	Mathematics Disorder
315.2	Disorder of Written Expression
315.31	Expressive Language Disorder
315.32	Mixed Receptive-Expressive Language Disorder
315.39	Phonological Disorder
315.4	Developmental Coordination Disorder
315.9	Learning Disorder NOS
316	. . . [Specified Psychological Factor] Affecting . . . [Indicate the General Medical Condition]
317	Mild Mental Retardation
318.0	Moderate Mental Retardation
318.1	Severe Mental Retardation
318.2	Profound Mental Retardation
319	Mental Retardation, Severity Unspecified
332.1	Neuroleptic-Induced Parkinsonism
333.1	Medication-Induced Postural Tremor
333.7	Neuroleptic-Induced Acute Dystonia
333.82	Neuroleptic-Induced Tardive Dyskinesia
333.90	Medication-Induced Movement Disorder NOS
333.92	Neuroleptic Malignant Syndrome
333.99	Neuroleptic-Induced Acute Akathisia
347	Narcolepsy
607.84	Male Erectile Disorder Due to . . . [Indicate the General Medical Condition]
608.89	Male Dyspareunia Due to . . . [Indicate the General Medical Condition]
608.89	Male Hypoactive Sexual Desire Disorder Due to . . . [Indicate the Medical Condition]
608.89	Other Male Sexual Dysfunction Due to . . . [Indicate the General Medical Condition]
625.0	Female Dyspareunia Due to . . . [Indicate the General Medical Condition]
625.8	Female Hypoactive Sexual Desire Disorder Due to . . . [Indicate the General Medical Condition]
625.8	Other Female Sexual Dysfunction Due to . . . [Indicate the General Medical Condition]
780.09	Delirium NOS

780.52   Sleep Disorder Due to . . . *[Indicate the General Medical Condition]*,
            Insomnia Type
780.54   Sleep Disorder Due to . . . *[Indicate the General Medical Condition]*,
            Hypersomnia Type
780.59   Breathing-Related Sleep Disorder
780.59   Sleep Disorder Due to . . . *[Indicate the General Medical Condition]*,
            Mixed Type
780.59   Sleep Disorder Due to . . . *[Indicate the General Medical Condition]*,
            Parasomnia Type
780.9   Age-Related Cognitive Decline
787.6   Encopresis, With Constipation and Overflow Incontinence
799.9   Diagnosis Deferred on Axis II
799.9   Diagnosis or Condition Deferred on Axis I
995.2   Adverse Effects of Medication NOS
995.52   Neglect of Child *(if focus of attention is on victim)*
995.53   Sexual Abuse of Child *(if focus of attention is on victim)*
995.54   Physical Abuse of Child *(if focus of attention is on victim)*
995.81   Physical Abuse of Adult *(if focus of attention is on victim)*
995.83   Sexual Abuse of Adult *(if focus of attention is on victim)*
V15.81   Noncompliance With Treatment
V61.10   Partner Relational Problem
V61.12   Physical Abuse of Adult (if by partner)
V61.12   Sexual Abuse of Adult (if by partner)
V61.20   Parent-Child Relational Problem
V61.21   Neglect of Child
V61.21   Physical Abuse of Child
V61.21   Sexual Abuse of Child
V61.8   Sibling Relational Problem
V61.9   Relational Problem Related to a Mental Disorder or
            General Medical Condition
V62.2   Occupational Problem
V62.3   Academic Problem
V62.4   Acculturation Problem
V62.81   Relational Problem NOS
V62.82   Bereavement
V62.83   Physical Abuse of Adult (if by person other than partner)
V62.83   Sexual Abuse of Adult (if by person other than partner)
V62.89   Borderline Intellectual Functioning
V62.89   Phase of Life Problem
V62.89   Religious or Spiritual Problem
V65.2   Malingering
V71.01   Adult Antisocial Behavior
V71.02   Child or Adolescent Antisocial Behavior
V71.09   No Diagnosis on Axis II
V71.09   No Diagnosis or Condition on Axis I

Appendix G

ICD-9-CM Codes for Selected General Medical Conditions and Medication-Induced Disorders

Updated to include ICD-9-CM codes effective October 1, 1996

The official coding system in use as of the publication of DSM-IV is the *International Classification of Diseases,* 9th Revision, Clinical Modification (ICD-9-CM). This appendix contains two sections that are provided to facilitate ICD-9-CM coding: 1) codes for selected general medical conditions, and 2) codes for medication-induced disorders.

ICD-9-CM Codes for Selected General Medical Conditions

The codes specified for use on Axis I and Axis II of DSM-IV represent only a small fraction of the codes provided in ICD-9-CM. The conditions classified outside the "Mental Disorders" chapter of ICD-9-CM are also important for clinical diagnosis and management in mental health settings. Axis III is provided to facilitate the reporting of these conditions (see DSM-IV p. 27). To assist clinicians in finding the ICD-9-CM codes, this appendix provides a selective index of those ICD-9-CM codes for general medical conditions that are most relevant to diagnosis and care in mental health settings. ICD-9-CM offers diagnostic specificity beyond that reflected in many of the codes that appear in this appendix (e.g., to denote a specific anatomical site or the presence of a specific complication). In cases in which increased specificity is noted in the fifth digit of the code, the least specific code (usually "0") has been selected. For example, the code for lymphosarcoma is given as 200.10 (for unspecified site), although more specificity with regard to anatomical site can be noted in the other fifth-digit codes, for example, 200.12 lymphosarcoma, intrathoracic lymph nodes. In cases in which increased specificity is reflected in the fourth digit of the code, this appendix often provides the "unspecified" category (e.g., 555.9 is listed for regional enteritis; ICD-9-CM also includes 555.0 for enteritis involving the small intestine, 555.1 for involvement of the large intestine, and 555.2 for involvement of both). Diagnostic codes for which more specificity is available are indicated in this appendix by an asterisk (*). Clinicians interested in recording greater specificity should refer to the complete listing of codes published in the ICD-9-CM Diseases: Tabular List (Volume 1) and the ICD-9-CM Diseases: Alphabetic Index (Volume 2). These documents are updated every October and are published by the U.S. Department of Health and Human Services. They are available from the Superintendent of Documents, U.S. Government Printing Office, as well as from a number of private publishers.

> **Note:** An asterisk (*) following the ICD-9-CM code indicates that greater specificity (e.g., a specific complication or anatomical site) is available. Refer to the ICD-9-CM Diseases: Tabular List (Volume 1) entry for that code for additional information.

Diseases of the Nervous System

324.0	Abscess, intracranial
331.0	Alzheimer's disease
437.0	Atherosclerosis, cerebral
354.0	Carpal tunnel syndrome
354.4	Causalgia
334.3	Cerebellar ataxia
850.9*	Concussion
851.80*	Contusion, cerebral
359.1	Dystrophy, Duchenne's muscular
348.5	Edema, cerebral
049.9*	Encephalitis, viral
572.2	Encephalopathy, hepatic
437.2	Encephalopathy, hypertensive
348.3*	Encephalopathy, unspecified
345.10*	Epilepsy, grand mal
345.40*	Epilepsy, partial, with impairment of consciousness (temporal lobe)
345.50*	Epilepsy, partial, without impairment of consciousness (Jacksonian)
345.00*	Epilepsy, petit mal (absences)
346.20	Headache, cluster
432.0	Hemorrhage, extradural, nontraumatic
852.40*	Hemorrhage, extradural, traumatic
431	Hemorrhage, intracerebral, nontraumatic
430	Hemorrhage, subarachnoid, nontraumatic
852.00*	Hemorrhage, subarachnoid, traumatic
432.1	Hemorrhage, subdural, nontraumatic
852.20*	Hemorrhage, subdural, traumatic
333.4	Huntington's chorea
331.3	Hydrocephalus, communicating
331.4	Hydrocephalus, obstructive
435.9*	Ischemic attack, transient
046.1	Creutzfeldt-Jakob disease
046.0	Kuru
046.3	Leukoencephalopathy, progressive multifocal
330.1	Lipidosis, cerebral
320.9*	Meningitis, bacterial (due to unspecified bacterium)
321.0	Meningitis, cryptococcal
054.72	Meningitis, herpes simplex virus
053.0	Meningitis, herpes zoster
321.1*	Meningitis, other fungal
094.2	Meningitis, syphilitic
047.9*	Meningitis, viral (due to unspecified virus)

346.00[*]   Migraine, classical (with aura)
346.10[*]   Migraine, common
346.90[*]   Migraine, unspecified
358.0   Myasthenia gravis
350.1   Neuralgia, trigeminal
337.1   Neuropathy, peripheral autonomic
434.9[*]   Occlusion, cerebral artery
350.2   Pain, face, atypical
351.0   Palsy, Bell's
343.9[*]   Palsy, cerebral
335.23   Palsy, pseudobulbar
046.2   Panencephalitis, subacute sclerosing
094.1   Paresis, general
332.0   Parkinson's disease, primary
331.1   Pick's disease
357.9[*]   Polyneuropathy
348.2   Pseudotumor cerebri (benign intracranial hypertension)
335.20   Sclerosis, amyotrophic lateral
340   Sclerosis, multiple (MS)
345.3   Status, grand mal
345.2   Status, petit mal
345.70   Status, temporal lobe
433.1   Stenosis, carotid artery, without cerebral infarction
436   Stroke (CVA)
330.1   Tay-Sachs disease
333.1   Tremor, benign essential

Diseases of the Circulatory System

413.9[*]   Angina pectoris
424.1   Aortic valve disorder
440.9[*]   Atherosclerosis
414.00[*]   Atherosclerotic heart disease
426.10[*]   Block, atrioventricular
426.3[*]   Block, left bundle branch
426.4   Block, right bundle branch
427.5   Cardiac arrest
425.5   Cardiomyopathy, alcoholic
425.4[*]   Cardiomyopathy, idiopathic
416.9[*]   Chronic pulmonary heart disease
427.9[*]   Dysrhythmia, cardiac, unspecified
415.19[*]   Embolism, pulmonary
421.9[*]   Endocarditis, bacterial
428.0[*]   Failure, congestive heart
427.31   Fibrillation, atrial
427.41   Fibrillation, ventricular
427.32   Flutter, atrial
427.42   Flutter, ventricular
455.6[*]   Hemorrhoids
401.9[*]   Hypertension, essential

402.91[*]   Hypertensive heart disease with congestive heart failure
402.90[*]   Hypertensive heart disease without congestive heart failure
403.91[*]   Hypertensive renal disease with failure
403.90[*]   Hypertensive renal disease without failure
458.0   Hypotension, orthostatic
410.90[*]   Infarction, myocardial, acute
424.0   Mitral valve insufficiency (nonrheumatic)
424.0   Mitral valve prolapse
394.0[*]   Mitral valve stenosis (rheumatic)
423.9[*]   Pericarditis
443.9[*]   Peripheral vascular disease
451.9[*]   Phlebitis/thrombophlebitis
446.0   Polyarteritis nodosa
427.60[*]   Premature beats
424.3   Pulmonary valve disease (nonrheumatic)
397.1   Pulmonary valve disease, rheumatic
427.0   Tachycardia, paroxysmal supraventricular
427.2   Tachycardia, paroxysmal, unspecified
427.1   Tachycardia, ventricular (paroxysmal)
424.2   Tricuspid valve disease (nonrheumatic)
397.0   Tricuspid valve disease, rheumatic
456.0   Varices, esophageal, with bleeding
456.1   Varices, esophageal, without bleeding
454.9[*]   Varicose veins, lower extremities

Diseases of the Respiratory System

513.0   Abscess of lung
518.0   Atelectasis
493.20[*]   Asthma, chronic obstructive
493.90[*]   Asthma, unspecified
494   Bronchiectasis
466.0   Bronchitis, acute
491.21   Bronchitis, obstructive chronic (COPD), with acute exacerbation
491.20   Bronchitis, obstructive chronic (COPD), without acute exacerbation
277.00[*]   Cystic fibrosis
511.9[*]   Effusion, pleural
492.8[*]   Emphysema
518.81[*]   Failure, respiratory
505   Pneumoconiosis
860.4[*]   Pneumohemothorax, traumatic
483.0   Pneumonia, mycoplasma
482.9[*]   Pneumonia, unspecified bacterial
481   Pneumonia, pneumococcal
136.3   Pneumonia, pneumocystis
482.30[*]   Pneumonia, streptococcus
486[*]   Pneumonia, unspecified organism
480.9[*]   Pneumonia, viral
512.8[*]   Pneumothorax, spontaneous
860.0[*]   Pneumothorax, traumatic
011.9[*]   Tuberculosis, pulmonary

Neoplasms

ICD-9-CM diagnostic codes for neoplasms are classified in the table of neoplasms in the ICD-9-CM Alphabetic Index (Volume 2) according to site and degree of malignancy (primary, secondary, in situ, benign, uncertain, unspecified).   **Note:** For patients with a personal history of malignant neoplasms that have been surgically removed or eradicated by chemotherapy or radiation therapy, codes V10.0–V10.9 should be used; for specific sites, refer to the Alphabetic Index (Volume 2) of ICD-9-CM under "History (personal) of, malignant neoplasm."

Listed below are some of the most common codes assigned for neoplasms.

228.02	Hemangioma of brain
201.90*	Hodgkin's disease
176.9*	Kaposi's sarcoma
208.01*	Leukemia, acute, in remission
208.00*	Leukemia, acute
208.11*	Leukemia, chronic, in remission
208.10*	Leukemia, chronic
200.10*	Lymphosarcoma
225.2	Meningioma (cerebral)
203.01	Multiple myeloma, in remission
203.00	Multiple myeloma
225.0	Neoplasm, benign, of brain
211.4	Neoplasm, benign, of colon
195.2	Neoplasm, malignant, abdominal cavity, primary
194.0	Neoplasm, malignant, adrenal gland, primary
188.9*	Neoplasm, malignant, bladder, primary
170.9*	Neoplasm, malignant, bone, primary
198.5	Neoplasm, malignant, bone, secondary
191.9*	Neoplasm, malignant, brain, primary
198.3	Neoplasm, malignant, brain, secondary
174.9*	Neoplasm, malignant, breast, female, primary
175.9*	Neoplasm, malignant, breast, male, primary
162.9*	Neoplasm, malignant, bronchus, primary
180.9*	Neoplasm, malignant, cervix, primary
153.9*	Neoplasm, malignant, colon, primary
197.5	Neoplasm, malignant, colon, secondary
171.9*	Neoplasm, malignant, connective tissue, primary
150.9*	Neoplasm, malignant, esophagus, primary
152.9*	Neoplasm, malignant, intestine, small, primary
189.0*	Neoplasm, malignant, kidney, primary
155.0	Neoplasm, malignant, liver, primary
197.7	Neoplasm, malignant, liver, secondary
162.9*	Neoplasm, malignant, lung, primary
197.0	Neoplasm, malignant, lung, secondary
196.9*	Neoplasm, malignant, lymph nodes, secondary
172.9*	Neoplasm, malignant, melanoma, primary
183.0*	Neoplasm, malignant, ovary, primary
157.9*	Neoplasm, malignant, pancreas, primary
185	Neoplasm, malignant, prostate, primary
154.1	Neoplasm, malignant, rectum, primary
173.9*	Neoplasm, malignant, skin, primary

151.9[*]   Neoplasm, malignant, stomach, site unspecified, primary
186.9[*]   Neoplasm, malignant, testis, primary
193   Neoplasm, malignant, thyroid, primary
179[*]   Neoplasm, malignant, uterus, primary
237.70[*]   Neurofibromatosis
227.0   Pheochromocytoma, benign
194.0   Pheochromocytoma, malignant
238.4   Polycythemia vera

Endocrine Diseases

253.0   Acromegaly
255.2   Adrenogenital disorder
259.2   Carcinoid syndrome
255.4   Corticoadrenal insufficiency
255.0   Cushing's syndrome
253.5   Diabetes insipidus
250.00[*]   Diabetes mellitus, type II/non-insulin-dependent
250.01[*]   Diabetes mellitus, type I/insulin-dependent
253.2   Dwarfism, pituitary
241.9[*]   Goiter, nontoxic nodular
240.9[*]   Goiter, simple
255.1   Hyperaldosteronism
252.0   Hyperparathyroidism
252.1   Hypoparathyroidism
244.9[*]   Hypothyroidism, acquired
243   Hypothyroidism, congenital
256.9[*]   Ovarian dysfunction
253.2   Panhypopituitarism
259.0   Sexual development and puberty, delayed
259.1   Sexual development and puberty, precocious
257.9[*]   Testicular dysfunction
245.9[*]   Thyroiditis
242.9[*]   Thyrotoxicosis

Nutritional Diseases

265.0   Beriberi
269.3   Calcium deficiency
266.2   Folic acid deficiency
269.3   Iodine deficiency
260   Kwashiorkor
262   Malnutrition, protein-caloric, severe
261   Nutritional marasmus
278.00[*]   Obesity
265.2   Pellagra (niacin deficiency)
266.0   Riboflavin deficiency
264.9[*]   Vitamin A deficiency
266.1   Vitamin B_6 deficiency
266.2   Vitamin B_{12} deficiency

267   Vitamin C deficiency
268.9*   Vitamin D deficiency
269.1   Vitamin E deficiency
269.0   Vitamin K deficiency

Metabolic Diseases

276.2   Acidosis
276.3   Alkalosis
277.3   Amyloidosis
276.5   Depletion, volume (dehydration)
271.3   Disaccharide malabsorption (lactose intolerance)
276.9*   Electrolyte imbalance
276.6   Fluid overload/retention
274.9*   Gout
275.0   Hemochromatosis
275.4   Hypercalcemia
276.7   Hyperkalemia
276.0   Hypernatremia
275.4   Hypocalcemia
276.8   Hypokalemia
276.1   Hyponatremia
270.1   Phenylketonuria (PKU)
277.1   Porphyria
277.2   Lesch-Nyhan syndrome
275.1   Wilson's disease

Diseases of the Digestive System

540.9*   Appendicitis, acute
578.9*   Bleeding, gastrointestinal
575.0   Cholecystitis, acute
575.11   Cholecystitis, chronic
571.2   Cirrhosis, alcoholic
556.9*   Colitis, ulcerative
564.0   Constipation
555.9*   Crohn's disease
009.2   Diarrhea, infectious
558.9*   Diarrhea, unspecified
562.10   Diverticulitis of colon, unspecified
562.12   Diverticulitis of colon, with hemorrhage
562.11   Diverticulosis of colon, unspecified
562.13   Diverticulosis of colon, with hemorrhage
535.50*   Duodenitis and gastritis
555.9*   Enteritis, regional
535.50*   Gastritis and duodenitis
558.9*   Gastroenteritis
530.1   Esophagitis
571.1   Hepatitis, alcoholic, acute
571.40*   Hepatitis, chronic

573.3*	Hepatitis, toxic (includes drug induced)
070.1*	Hepatitis, viral A
070.30*	Hepatitis, viral B
070.51*	Hepatitis, viral C
560.39*	Impaction, fecal
550.90*	Inguinal hernia
564.1	Irritable bowel syndrome
576.2	Obstruction, bile duct
560.9*	Obstruction, intestinal
577.0	Pancreatitis, acute
577.1	Pancreatitis, chronic
567.9*	Peritonitis
530.1	Reflux, esophageal
530.4	Rupture, esophageal
530.3	Stricture, esophageal
532.30*	Ulcer, duodenal, acute
532.70*	Ulcer, duodenal, chronic
531.30*	Ulcer, gastric, acute
531.70*	Ulcer, gastric, chronic

Genitourinary System Diseases

596.4	Atonic bladder
592.0	Calculus, renal
592.1	Calculus, ureter
592.9*	Calculus, urinary, unspecified
595.9*	Cystitis
625.3	Dysmenorrhea
617.9*	Endometriosis
584.9*	Failure, renal, acute
585	Failure, renal, chronic
403.91*	Failure, renal, hypertensive
586*	Failure, renal, unspecified
218.9*	Fibroid of uterus
580.9*	Glomerulonephritis, acute
600	Hypertrophy, prostatic, benign (BPH)
628.9*	Infertility, female
606.9*	Infertility, male
627.9*	Menopausal or postmenopausal disorder
626.9*	Menstruation, disorder of, and abnormal bleeding
625.2	Mittelschmerz
620.2*	Ovarian cyst
614.9*	Pelvic inflammatory disease (PID)
607.3	Priapism
618.9*	Prolapse, genital
601.9*	Prostatitis
593.3	Stricture, ureteral
598.9*	Stricture, urethral
599.0	Urinary tract infection (UTI)

Hematological Diseases

288.0	Agranulocytosis
287.0	Allergic purpura
284.9*	Anemia, aplastic
281.2	Anemia, folate-deficiency
283.9*	Anemia, hemolytic, acquired
283.11	Anemia, hemolytic-uremic syndrome
280.9*	Anemia, iron-deficiency
283.10	Anemia, nonautoimmune hemolytic, unspecified
283.19	Anemia, other autoimmune hemolytic
281.0	Anemia, pernicious
282.60*	Anemia, sickle-cell
286.9*	Coagulation defects
288.3	Eosinophilia
282.4	Thalassemia
287.5*	Thrombocytopenia

Diseases of the Eye

366.9*	Cataract
372.9*	Conjunctiva disorder
361.9*	Detachment, retinal
365.9*	Glaucoma
377.30*	Neuritis, optic
379.50*	Nystagmus
377.00*	Papilledema
369.9*	Visual loss

Diseases of the Ear, Nose, and Throat

460	Common cold
389.9*	Hearing loss
464.0	Laryngitis, acute
386.00*	Ménière's disease
382.9*	Otitis media
462	Pharyngitis, acute
477.9*	Rhinitis, allergic
461.9*	Sinusitis, acute
473.9*	Sinusitis, chronic
388.30*	Tinnitus, unspecified
463	Tonsillitis, acute

Musculoskeletal System and Connective Tissue Diseases

716.20*	Arthritis, allergic
711.90*	Arthritis, infective
714.0	Arthritis, rheumatoid
733.40*	Aseptic necrosis of bone
710.3	Dermatomyositis

722.91   Disc disorder, intervertebral, cervical
722.93   Disc disorder, intervertebral, lumbar
722.92   Disc disorder, intervertebral, thoracic
733.10*   Fracture, pathological
715.90*   Osteoarthrosis (osteoarthritis)
730.20*   Osteomyelitis
733.00*   Osteoporosis
710.1   Scleroderma (systemic sclerosis)
737.30   Scoliosis
710.2   Sjögren's disease
720.0   Spondylitis, ankylosing
710.0   Systemic lupus erythematosus

Diseases of the Skin

704.00*   Alopecia
692.9*   Dermatitis, contact
693.0*   Dermatitis, due to substance (taken internally)
682.9*   Cellulitis, unspecified site
695.1   Erythema multiforme
703.0   Ingrowing nail
701.4   Keloid scar
696.1*   Psoriasis
707.0   Ulcer, decubitus
708.0   Urticaria, allergic

Congenital Malformations, Deformations, and Chromosomal Abnormalities

749.10*   Cleft lip
749.00*   Cleft palate
758.3   Cri-du-chat syndrome (antimongolism)
758.0   Down's syndrome
760.71   Fetal alcohol syndrome
751.3   Hirschsprung's disease (congenital colon dysfunction)
742.3   Hydrocephalus, congenital
752.7   Indeterminate sex and pseudohermaphroditism
758.7   Klinefelter's syndrome
759.82   Marfan's syndrome
742.1   Microcephalus
741.90*   Spina bifida
750.5   Stenosis, congenital hypertrophic pyloric
760.71   Toxic effects of alcohol
760.75   Toxic effects of cocaine
760.73   Toxic effects of hallucinogens
760.72   Toxic effects of narcotics
760.70   Toxic effects of other substances (including medications)
759.5   Tuberous sclerosis
758.6   Turner's syndrome
752.51   Undescended testicle

Diseases of Pregnancy, Childbirth, and the Puerperium

Diagnoses associated with pregnancies can be located in the Alphabetic Index (Volume 2) of ICD-9-CM indented under "Pregnancy, complicated (by)," or "Pregnancy, management affected by." Listed below are some of the most common conditions.

642.00*	Eclampsia
643.0*	Hyperemesis gravidarum, mild
643.0*	Hyperemesis gravidarum, with metabolic disturbance
642.0*	Pre-eclampsia, mild
642.0*	Pre-eclampsia, severe

Infectious Diseases

The following codes represent ICD-9-CM diagnostic codes for infections from specific organisms. Traditionally, codes for organisms from the 041 category are used as secondary codes (e.g., urinary tract infection due to *Escherichia coli* would be coded as 599.0 [primary diagnosis] and 041.4 [secondary diagnosis]).

006.9*	Amebiasis
112.5	Candidiasis, disseminated
112.4	Candidiasis, lung
112.0	Candidiasis, mouth
112.2	Candidiasis, other urogenital sites
112.3	Candidiasis, skin and nails
112.9	Candidiasis, unspecified site
112.1	Candidiasis, vulva and vagina
099.41	*Chlamydia trachomatis*
001.9*	Cholera
041.83	*Clostridium perfrigens*
114.9*	Coccidioidomycosis
078.1	*Condyloma acuminatum* (viral warts)
079.2	Coxsackie virus
117.5	Cryptococcosis
041.4	*Escherichia coli (E. coli)*
007.1	Giardiasis
098.2*	Gonorrhea
041.5	*Hemophilus influenzae (H. influenzae)*
070.1*	Hepatitis, viral A
070.3*	Hepatitis, viral B
070.51	Hepatitis, viral C
054.9*	Herpes simplex
053.9*	Herpes zoster
115.9*	Histoplasmosis
042	HIV infection (symptomatic)
036.9*	Infection, meningococcal
079.99*	Infection, viral, unspecified
487.1	Influenza, unspecified
487.0	Influenza, with pneumonia
041.3*	*Klebsiella pneumoniae*
088.81	Lyme disease
084.6*	Malaria

075	Mononucleosis
072.9*	Mumps
041.81	*Mycoplasma*
041.2	*Pneumococcus*
041.6	*Proteus*
041.7	*Pseudomonas*
071	Rabies
056.9*	Rubella
003.9*	Salmonella
135	Sarcoidosis
004.9*	Shigellosis
041.10*	*Staphylococcus*
041.00*	*Streptococcus*
097.9*	Syphilis
082.9*	Tick-borne rikettsiosis
130.9*	Toxoplasmosis
124	Trichinosis
131.9*	Trichomoniasis
002.0	Typhoid fever
081.9*	Typhus

Overdose

Additional diagnostic codes for overdose/poisoning can be located in the Alphabetic Index (Volume 2) of ICD-9-CM in the table of drugs and chemicals, listed alphabetically by drug in the "Poisoning" column.

965.4	Acetaminophen
962.0	Adrenal cortical steroids
972.4	Amyl/butyl/nitrite
962.1	Androgens and anabolic steroids
971.1	Anticholinergics
969.0	Antidepressants
967.0	Barbiturates
969.4	Benzodiazepine-based tranquilizers
969.2	Butyrophenone-based tranquilizers
967.1	Chloral hydrate
968.5	Cocaine
967.5	Glutethimide
969.6	Hallucinogens/cannabis
962.3	Insulin and antidiabetic agents
967.4	Methaqualone
968.2	Nitrous oxide
970.1	Opioid antagonists
965.00	Opioids
967.2	Paraldehyde
968.3	Phencyclidine
969.1	Phenothiazine-based tranquilizers
965.1	Salicylates
970.9	Stimulants
962.7	Thyroid and thyroid derivatives

Additional Codes for Medication-Induced Disorders

The following are the ICD-9-CM codes for selected medications that may cause Substance-Induced Disorders. They are made available for optional use by clinicians in situations in which these medications, prescribed at therapeutic dose levels, have resulted in one of the following: Substance-Induced Delirium, Substance-Induced Persisting Dementia, Substance-Induced Persisting Amnestic Disorder, Substance-Induced Psychotic Disorder, Substance-Induced Mood Disorder, Substance-Induced Anxiety Disorder, Substance-Induced Sexual Dysfunction, Substance-Induced Sleep Disorder, and Medication-Induced Movement Disorders. When used in multiaxial evaluation, the E-codes should be coded on Axis I immediately following the related disorder. It should be noted that these E-codes do not apply to poisonings or to a medication taken as an overdose.

Example: 292.39   Substance-Induced Mood Disorder, With Depressive Features
E932.2   Oral contraceptives

Analgesics and Antipyretics

E935.4   Acetaminophen/phenacetin
E935.1   Methadone
E935.6   Nonsteroidal anti-inflammatory agents
E935.2   Other narcotics (e.g., codeine, meperidine)
E935.3   Salicylates (e.g., aspirin)

Anticonvulsants

E936.3   Carbamazepine
E936.2   Ethosuximide
E937.0   Phenobarbital
E936.1   Phenytoin
E936.3   Valproic acid

Antiparkinsonian Medications

E936.4   Amantadine
E941.1   Benztropine
E933.0   Diphenhydramine
E936.4   L-Dopa

Neuroleptic Medications

E939.2   Butyrophenone-based neuroleptics (e.g., haloperidol)
E939.3   Other neuroleptics (e.g., thiothixene)
E939.1   Phenothiazine-based neuroleptics (e.g., chlorpromazine)

Sedatives, Hypnotics, and Anxiolytics

E937.0   Barbiturates
E939.4   Benzodiazepine-based medications
E937.1   Chloral hydrate
E939.5   Hydroxyzine
E937.2   Paraldehyde

Other Psychotropic Medications

E939.0   Antidepressants
E939.6   Cannabis
E940.1   Opioid antagonists
E939.7   Stimulants (excluding central appetite depressants)

Cardiovascular Medications

E942.0   Antiarrhythmic medication (includes propranolol)
E942.2   Antilipemic and cholesterol-lowering medication
E942.1   Cardiac glycosides (e.g., digitalis)
E942.4   Coronary vasodilators (e.g., nitrates)
E942.3   Ganglion-blocking agents (pentamethonium)
E942.6   Other antihypertensive agents (e.g., clonidine, guanethidine, reserpine)
E942.5   Other vasodilators (e.g., hydralazine)

Primarily Systemic Agents

E933.0   Antiallergic and antiemetic agents (excluding phenothiazines, hydroxyzine)
E941.1   Anticholinergics (e.g., atropine) and spasmolytics
E934.2   Anticoagulants
E933.1   Antineoplastic and immunosuppressive drugs
E941.0   Cholinergics (parasympathomimetics)
E941.2   Sympathomimetics (adrenergics)
E933.5   Vitamins (excluding vitamin K)

Medications Acting on Muscles and the Respiratory System

E945.7   Antiasthmatics (aminophylline)
E945.4   Antitussives (e.g., dextromethorphan)
E945.8   Other respiratory drugs
E945.0   Oxytocic agents (ergot alkaloids, prostaglandins)
E945.2   Skeletal muscle relaxants
E945.1   Smooth muscle relaxants (metaproterenol)

Hormones and Synthetic Substitutes

E932.0   Adrenal cortical steroids
E932.1   Anabolic steroids and androgens
E932.8   Antithyroid agents
E932.2   Ovarian hormones (includes oral contraceptives)
E932.7   Thyroid replacements

Diuretics and Mineral and Uric Acid Metabolism Drugs

E944.2   Carbonic acid anhydrase inhibitors
E944.3   Chlorthiazides
E944.0   Mercurial diuretics
E944.4   Other diuretics (furosemide, ethacrynic acid)
E944.1   Purine derivative diuretics
E944.7   Uric acid metabolism drugs (probenecid)